Just Briefly

From the Chief Medical Officer

One of my most important roles over the last three years has been as a member of the Executive Board of the World Health Organization (WHO), which advises the WHO's Director General, and through him the World Health Assembly, on matters related to improving health for all[1]. In January, the third Report entitled *Monitoring of Progress and Implementation of Strategies for Health For all by the Year 2000* was presented. It summarised progress in this global strategy for health for all during 1991-93. A total of 131 member states with a population of 4,841 million reported their findings in time for analysis. The results are fascinating and I can only, in this editorial, give a few of the relevant figures.

For example, the global target for life expectancy adopted in 1981 was to exceed 60 years in every country of the world by the year 2000. Overall life expectancy has increased, but there are still 26 developing countries (with 10% of the world's population) which have a life expectancy at birth of less than 60 years. On average, women live seven years longer than men in developed countries and three years longer in developing countries.

Infant mortality is still a challenge. In the European region, for example, infant mortality continues to fall but disparities persist and are even increasing in some of the newly independent states. Maternal mortality rates world wide range from approximately 530 per 100,000 live births in the least developed countries to less than 10 per 100,000 in developed countries.

Almost half of all deaths are directly related to an infectious or parasitic disease. There is a clear contrast between developed countries, where communicable diseases in children are generally controlled and the vast majority of deaths occur later in life (with almost three-quarters occurring after the age of 65 years), and developing countries at the first stage of development in which over one-third of deaths occur below the age of 5 years, one-third between 5 and 64 years, and the remainder after the age of 65. The figures for communicable diseases are striking. For example, almost 40% of the population of the world is exposed to malaria to some degree. In sub-Saharan Africa it is estimated that there are between 270 and 480 million clinical cases of malaria per year, with 1.4 to 2.8 million deaths. Many communicable diseases are preventable by vaccination, and a general decline has been seen thanks to the progress made by the expanded programme on immunisation. For polio, 141 countries reported no cases in 1993. In Europe, however, there were two major epidemics in Azerbaijan and Uzbekistan in 1993. Endemic transmission of polio appears to have ceased in the Americas, where no cases of the disease due to a wild virus has been detected since 1991.

Most strikingly, over one third of the world's population is now infected with *Mycobacterium tuberculosis*. There are approximately 8 million new cases each year, 7.6 million of them in developing countries, and almost 3 million deaths. The link between tuberculosis and HIV infection is well recorded world wide. More than 18 million adults and 1 million children have contracted HIV since the start of the epidemic, with 80-90% of childhood infections occurring in sub-Saharan Africa. The global annual incidence of sexually transmitted disease other than AIDS is estimated at 250 million cases, predominantly in developing countries. The number of cases of leprosy in the world fell to 2.4 million in 1994, compared with 5.5 million in 1991 (when the target for elimination of this disease with multidrug therapy was set for the year 2000).

Non-communicable diseases account for at least 40% of deaths in developing and 75% in industrialised countries. For example, diabetes mellitus affects at least 60 million adults including 2-5% of adults in Europe, and is increasing in developing countries in relation to changes in lifestyle. Injury and violence still constitute a persistent problem especially in young people in most countries. The report points out that there are least 300 million suffering from some sort of mental or neurological illness. Disability is also increasing.

This brief account of some indicators of health status show how far we have come, but also how far we still have to go: attaining health for all will not be easy, but it is a goal to be strived for.

On a quite different note I recently visited Helen House in Oxford which, when it opened in 1982, was the first children's hospice in the United Kingdom (UK). I had an interesting discussion about the work of the hospice and its role in the care of children with a life-limiting illness with Mary Thompson, the Head Nurse, Sister Frances Dominica, the hospice's founder, Dr Hilary Allinson, one of the local general practitioners (GPs) who provide medical cover, and Richard and Jacqueline Worswick, whose daughter Helen was the inspiration behind the hospice. I also had the chance to talk to members of the care team and see the work of the hospice at first hand.

Helen House is a small, eight-bedded, purpose-built unit set in a beautiful garden. The hospice provides respite and terminal care for children with a life-limiting illness and support for their families. Since the children who come to Helen House are primarily cared for at home, the model for the hospice is the family home. The emphasis is on helping each child, within the limitations imposed by his or her condition to live life to the full, if not in terms of length at least in terms of quality.

Since it opened over 300 children from all over the UK have used Helen House. Of these over half have come from within a 50 mile radius of Oxford although some come from considerably further afield. There is also accommodation for families which is currently being extended. Though the length of visits varies, most are of less than one week's duration. Initial inquiries about what the hospice might be able to offer come from the family itself or from someone involved in a professional capacity - a GP, consultant, social worker or teacher. Children are not normally taken for the first time over the age of 16 years. There are no fees; Helen House is funded entirely by charitable donations.

Across the region in Cambridgeshire, I visited Hinchbrook Health Care Trust mental health service in Park House, a facility located in the centre of Huntingdon, which provides a 35-place day service and a base for three community mental health teams covering this rural area. The day service caters for people with severe and long-term mental illness, and also those in crisis needing intensive support. The day service provides an active rehabilitation programme and links people into work opportunities. One example of this is the snack bar project which provides catering for Park House and adjoining health service facilities. There are a number of innovative therapeutic projects, such as an early intervention programme for people with psychosis, to enable them to take more control in managing their illness. More extensive out-of-hours provision will further help to develop the intensive support service as an alternative to admission.

Multidisciplinary team work forms the basis of the clinical work, with good working relation between health and social services. This style of working is also evident in other aspects of service delivery. The Care Programme Approach has been successfully implemented and integrated with care management. This process has been important in targeting resources to the severely mentally ill. Use of one set of case notes per patient may appear to be a small and obvious issue, but it is not achieved in all mental health services and has been very important in improving communication and patient care. An integrated information system has been developed so that all patient contacts with the mental health services are consistently recorded and provide a patient register and database which is used in workload management, clinical audit and outcome research.

I also visited the Mitchell Day Centre, part of the Cambridgeshire Psychiatric Rehabilitation Service (CPRS), which was designated as a national demonstration centre in February 1989 and has been in the forefront of providing care for long-term seriously mentally ill patients for nearly three decades, including those living in the community. More recently, the appointment of a consultant with special interest in research and treatment of schizophrenia has added yet another dimension to the sophistication of the service.

The CPRS supports 170 clients in the community, 110 of whom attend Mitchell Day Centre. The rest are supported in their homes by community psychiatric nurses, occupational therapists and day-support workers from social services. Mitchell Day Centre has recently moved from Fulbourn Hospital to newly refurbished

accommodation in the city. The centre offers a variety of therapeutic programmes specifically targeted to the most disabled of clients, 70% of whom have schizophrenia; it also runs a depot clinic and a clozapine clinic. The clients get lunch, perhaps the only hot meal for many of them. Further services include daily visits by the medical staff who also hold a fortnightly clinic. Perhaps the uniqueness of the centre lies in its ambience of hospitality and informality calculated to attract those who are most disorganised and difficult to engage. It demonstrated just what a remarkable challenge there is in community nursing.

Finally, Yaxley group practice and the Yaxley Health Centre Patients' Association. Yaxley group practice is a semi-rural practice with approximately 11,500 patients, some 5,000 living in the surrounding villages with little or no public transport. The Patients' Association was formed following pressure from the practice and local parish councils to improve transport facilities for the patients, which resulted in a special dial-a-bus service. The first annual general meeting was held in 1984, a constitution drawn up and a logo designed by local schoolchildren. As well as raising well over £20,000 to purchase equipment, one of the main priorities of the Association has been health education. All patients are automatically members of the Association and the committee is made up of representatives from all the villages covered by the practice. In 1991 the Association decided to establish a patients' library and resource centre; a librarian who had trained with the Citizens Advice Bureau was appointed, initially for 5 hours a week, and was also able to offer advice on benefit and housing matters. Plans are now being made for a pilot project involving the use of shared records with patients, beginning with the chronically ill housebound patients and those in residential homes. The Association, together with their health promotion unit are holding a resources exhibition for parents of young people aged 10 to 16 years when there will be an opportunity to talk about some of the difficulties experienced by parents and teenagers.

Kenneth C. Calman

References

1 *Primary health care: report of the International Conference on Primary Health Care, Alma-Ata 1978.* Geneva: World Health Organization, 1978. (Health for All series; No.1).

2 World Health Organization. *Monitoring of progress in implementation of strategies for health for all by the year 2000: third Report.* Geneva: WHO, 1994.

Editorials

Trends in *Health Trends*

The Editorial Board spends much time reviewing *Health Trends'* publishing policy to ensure that it continues to meet the remit set for us by Sir George Godber[1]. As the structure and needs of the Department of Health (DH) and National Health Service (NHS) develop, so we have to change our scope. What then are our present objectives? Our guidelines at present are broad - "medical aspects of NHS practice, management, planning, implementation and evaluation". Within that canvas we lay great emphasis on innovation, monitoring, audit and an epidemiological approach. Our recent review article, by Professor Harry Keen on the Diabetes Control and Complications Trial (DCCT)[2], was a new venture to present important clinical developments in a concise and authoritative form.

After review, it has been suggested that these objectives be more clearly defined, and could be summarised as to provide:

- the Chief Medical Officer and other chief professional officers with the opportunity to communicate directly and publicly with the medical profession on important topical items;

- clear statements on DH policies and initiatives;

- clear information on good clinical practice and clinical audit;

- space for original papers in relevant fields;

- a correspondence section to debate the scientific issues raised in our columns; *and*

- occasional commissioned review articles on important developments.

The Board is only too well aware that with our large readership we cannot satisfy everyone, but we hope that in every issue there are some contributions which each reader finds of interest and value. No doubt we could do better - but to do this the Board needs your help. I therefore invite readers with constructive views of the journal to write to me. Are we meeting our current objectives, and are we selecting the right sort of papers for publication after peer review? I would especially welcome views on the proposed changes to our publication policy. Having set it out, have we got it right? Even though we already have a heavy postbag, which I hope will enlarge following this plea, let me add that we greatly welcome receiving original articles, although currently only about one in ten submitted articles is chosen for publication.

I look forward to your response, so that as *Health Trends* enters its 26th year, the Board can decide how best to improve the service it provides to you, our readers, whilst preserving the journal's original function "...to provide a convenient vehicle for distribution in compact form of information bearing on the service and not otherwise readily available to the professions working in it".

Michael Abrams
Chairman, Editorial Board
c/o Room 104 Eileen House,
80-94 Newington Causeway,
London SE1 6EF

References
1 Godber G. Editorial. *Health Trends* 1969; **1:** 1.
2 Keen H. The Diabetes Control and Complications Trial (DCCT). *Health Trends* 1994; **26:** 41-3.

Editorial note: Retirement of Miss Julia Coon

Miss Julia Coon, Production Editor of *Health Trends*, retired from the Department of Health on 30 March 1995 after a long and distinguished career. The Editorial Board and her colleagues in the Editorial Unit thank Miss Coon for her sterling work on *Health Trends* and the Unit's other publications over many years, and wish her a long and happy retirement.

Use of Office of Population Censuses and Surveys records in medical research and clinical audit

Beverley Botting*, Statistician, **Harry Reilly**, Higher Executive Officer, Office of Population Censuses and Surveys (OPCS), St Catherine's House, 10 Kingsway London, WC2B 6JB, and **David Harris**, Higher Executive Officer, OPCS, Smedley Hydro, Trafalgar Road, Birkdale, Southport, PR8 2HH.

Keywords: Medical research; clinical audit; statistics; patient tracing.

Health Trends 1995; **27**: 4-7

Introduction

Clinicians and epidemiologists have become increasingly interested in access to patient records for clinical audit and medical research. This article describes the historical background of the Office of Population Censuses and Surveys (OPCS), and the ways in which its records can be used to support such research. It also discusses how confidentiality is safeguarded, whilst at the same time access for those with approved studies has been improved.

Background

"I requested permission . . . to take a list, at the General Register Office, of the deaths from cholera . . . in the subdistricts of Golden Square, Berwick Street and St. Ann's, Soho . . . which was kindly granted." [1]

Snow's 1849 report *On the mode of communication of cholera* was a model for future medical research using information from death certificates. When he discovered that this particular outbreak was confined to people who drank water from a certain pump-well:

"I had an interview with the Board of Guardians of St. James Parish . . . and in consequence of what I said the handle of the pump was removed on the following day."

Data from vital statistical records have been used for medical research purposes almost since civil registration began in England and Wales in 1837. At first, this simply allowed access to the non-confidential parts of vital registration documents to researchers outside the General Register Office (as it was known then - GRO changed its name to OPCS in 1970). Ad-hoc enquiries by registrars of deaths also proved effective:

"I have registered 50 deaths from smallpox from January 1st to June 30th, 1845; only one of the fifty persons had been vaccinated, and that was a doubtful case . . ." [2]

"Smallpox has appeared in part of my district. I find, on enquiry, that a vast number of parents have not availed themselves of vaccination." [2]

**Correspondent: Mrs B Botting

Medical research based only on information from death certificates then developed rapidly, enabling retrospective enquiries into specific causes. This was possible using 'death drafts', which are copies of the death entries submitted by registrars to the Registrar General. In the 1950s, Case and Hosker[3] examined a complete set of death drafts for bladder cancers from 1921 onwards, and found a marked excess among men who had been employed in the dyestuffs industry compared with the national average. Similarly, Doll and Bradford Hill received copies of death drafts relating to medical practitioners from 1952 onwards, which contributed to their important longitudinal study of smoking habits and the health of doctors[4].

The 1950s saw a rapid increase in the number of longitudinal studies of occupational health hazards. One of the early studies in which GRO traced individuals through the National Health Service Central Register (NHSCR) was the cohort of women who painted luminous paint onto watchfaces and were thought to be at particular risk of cancer[5]. Methods for tracing individuals in occupational studies were described by Newhouse and Williams[6] in their study of the health of individuals who had worked in an asbestos factory: they started by searching in the records kept by the then Ministry of Pensions and National Insurance for the names of employees, with the NHSCR used as a secondary source. It was also about this time that a way of marking ('flagging') the entry on the NHSCR of those traced was developed, so that death drafts could be supplied to the researchers for all subsequent deaths. A detailed historical account of past studies in occupational health using OPCS data has recently been published[7]. A list of all studies up to 1991 which have been helped by OPCS is given in the review of OPCS's medical research services by a working group of the Registrar General's Medical Advisory Committee[8].

OPCS' medical research services have been widely used in studies of the natural history of disease, and comparing prognoses after different treatment regimens - such as the Medical Research Council (MRC) trials of treatments for leukaemia[9], and collaborative international trials of thrombolytics in patients with suspected acute myocardial infarction.

Increased emphasis on clinical audit to identify factors which led to particular adverse outcomes has seen the establishment of various confidential enquiries into such adverse outcomes, and OPCS has been able to help by identifying deaths of interest to each enquiry.

OPCS

OPCS is a separate Government department formed in 1970 when the General Register Office (established 1837) merged with the Government Social Survey (started in 1941). It is a statutory body, with a duty to prepare and publish statistics about the number and condition of the population during periods between national censuses. OPCS is closely linked to the NHS because it maintains and processes several health information systems on behalf of the Department of Health (DH). Its main functions include:

collection of information from the public, for example through the registration of births, marriages and deaths;

the decennial census of population and ad-hoc social surveys;

processing cancer registrations, abortion notifications, congenital malformation notifications, and notifications of infectious diseases;

producing routine population and health statistics;

maintaining and administering the NHSCR and other registers;

storing data in a secure and retrievable form; *and*

making information available for customers.

Thus, OPCS holds considerable information about the health and circumstances of a large number of individuals, whilst protecting the confidentiality of the people to whom the information relates. OPCS retains anonymous abstracts to compile statistical reports, but can also extract information about identifiable individuals from key sources such as Censuses, vital registration records and cancer registers to help those involved in medical research.

Type of support for medical research

OPCS can help researchers in several ways: it can identify individuals who have died of particular causes, suffered from specific cancers, or who are at particular risk because of their occupation, or place of residence or birth; it can prospectively identify deaths of, or occurrence of cancer in, individuals identified by researchers as samples or particular medical cohorts of research interest; and can help with case-control studies, for example by providing data about study members and controls. For cohort studies, OPCS can help to document the survival or occurrence of cancer in study members, and compare these with population risks.

For some studies where the researcher has been given ethical approval to contact the cohort members or their medical attendants, an additional service of OPCS is to inform the researchers of the current Family Health Services Authority (FHSA) where the given individuals are registered with a general practitioner (GP). While OPCS does not hold any details about the individual's address, the FHSA will usually forward any letters from the researcher to the individual's GP.

OPCS can also help with more complex linkage studies, where the researcher may wish to contact, or find out, the status of relatives of cohort members. This could include bringing together information from across OPCS's record systems for the same individuals. For example, OPCS could identify relatives using the original 1939 NHSCR books which were grouped by households, or birth or marriage data, and then trace the current FHSA where study members are registered with an NHS GP.

Provision of death drafts

Death entries provide information about the deceased's age, occupation, where they lived and the conditions contributing to the death. By holding this data we can identify individuals who have died of particular causes and provide researchers with death drafts. For deaths after 28 days-of-age before 1993, and neonatal deaths before 1986, only the underlying cause was coded and held on the computer except for the years 1975/76 and 1985/86 when OPCS coded all conditions given on the certificate. Since 1986 for neonatal deaths and since 1993 for all deaths, all causes given on the death entries have been coded and held on the computer by OPCS.

For deaths occurring from 1993 onwards, computer programmes originally developed in the United States of America, and adapted by OPCS, are used to code cause of death automatically. By January 1995, 74% of all death entries were automatically coded.

Death drafts are used in various studies, ranging from small studies which request a copy of the death entry for deaths of named patients being studied by the researchers, to larger national, regional or cohort surveys of all deaths of a particular type. The completeness of ascertainment depends on how well the medical certificate of cause of death has been completed, as well as on the quality of searches at OPCS.

Use of birth drafts

Occasionally, researchers may wish to know the place of birth or other non-confidential particulars about the birth of given individuals, and OPCS will undertake to find and copy the relevant drafts for the researchers. Similarly, OPCS can provide non-confidential information about births occurring at a particular place or time.

Tracing and flagging studies

Where researchers wish to know the current status of individuals of particular interest to them, usually in a cohort at particular risk, OPCS can help by using the NHSCR to trace the individuals and note their current FHSA 'posting', or report an 'exit' from the register. Where there has been a death or a cancer marked against the entry, the researcher is sent a copy of the death and/or cancer draft retrospectively. As mentioned earlier, the entry can also be marked with the relevant medical research project number (known as 'flagging') so that the researcher can be informed of any subsequent death or cancer registration as soon as it is reported to NHSCR.

Some two million people are currently flagged in the NHSCR in over 420 separate studies - some broad groups of studies have

Table 1: *Number of flagged individuals in various studies*

Type of study	All	Number of flags								
		Under 100	100-999	1000-4999	5000-9999	10000-19999	20000-49999	50000-99999	100000 and over	Not stated
All studies	421	24	139	139	52	34	15	8	3	7
Studies of the effects of health hazards	136	5	30	56	22	8	7	6	1	1
Studies of effectiveness of therapy or screening	116	12	48	30	9	9	4	1	1	2
Health and behaviour survey and outcomes	48	2	12	16	6	6	3	1	1	1
Genetic studies	15	-	5	3	4	2	-	-	-	1
Studies of epidemiology and natural history of disease	105	5	43	34	11	9	1	-	-	2
Not stated	1	-	1	-	-	-	-	-	-	-

been described earlier in this article. Table 1 shows some types of study and the number of flagged individuals as at 30 June 1994.

Usually, cohort members have been identified by researchers outside OPCS. They include:

occupationally based cohorts, identified from employers' records;

cohort studies based on knowledge of behaviour, such as smoking, determined from a cross-sectional survey;

individuals diagnosed as having certain disorders such as Down's Syndrome, cerebral palsy or diabetes mellitus; *and*

those who have had a specific treatment or have been screened for a particular cancer.

Links with the Scottish Central Register
The England and Wales NHSCR holds an entry for each resident registered with an NHS GP in England and Wales. Similarly, the General Register Office (Scotland) Central Register covers those registered in Scotland, and there is routine exchange of information between these registers about flagged individuals. The Scottish NHSCR has been described by Hedley and McMaster[10].

Recent developments
Since 1 January 1991, a new computerised NHS Central Register has been compiled by aggregating the computer records of all FHSAs. It includes a record for all individuals in England and Wales alive on 1 January 1991, together with immigrants who have registered with an NHS GP, and all births since 1991. As far as possible all duplicate registrations have been removed, and mistakes corrected.

The new NHS computerised Register, the Central Health Register Inquiry System (CHRIS), contains flags relating to both cancer registration and those which indicate membership of any existing medical research study. Future flags will be added as required. For individuals on CHRIS, tracing and flagging activities are greatly simplified compared with the manual system.

Eventually, all registration offices of births, deaths and marriages will enter registration details directly onto a computer database.

By January 1995, this was the case for 87% of birth and death registrations. The electronic transfer of registration details to OPCS, including textual information not previously coded, began in January 1993. For births and deaths after January 1993, relevant draft entries can be selected and printed electronically, collapsing into one stage the processes of searching through indexes, then through microfiches of drafts, and then copying and printing the drafts. It is also possible to select the items to be released to the researchers electronically, thus avoiding the laborious task of masking confidential data before it can be copied.

Regional cancer registries send notifications to the OPCS national cancer system at Titchfield on magnetic tape, and within OPCS these data are subsequently transferred (again by magnetic tape), to the NHSCR. If the identification details are adequate, it is possible to merge directly cancer data with the NHSCR, and automatically flag the NHSCR computerised system; otherwise, computer-assisted searches have to be made.

During 1994, OPCS introduced a facility to transfer to NHSCR data on magnetic tape or floppy disk, which simplifies (and reduces the cost to medical researchers) flagging and event notification.

Future alternatives to flagging
Until now, requests for assistance from medical researchers have largely been confined to data needed for studies as described above - such as case-control and cohort studies involving requests for flagging or tracing to ascertain survival, cancer incidence, cause of death, or present whereabouts of the individual concerned. Increasingly, however, there is a requirement for large-scale tracing or flagging studies; sometimes for surveillance of possible effects of environmental hazards, such as radiation; sometimes to evaluate screening programmes, such as for cancers of the cervix, breast or colon; and sometimes to set up family studies. However, for some purposes it might become unnecessary to flag the CHRIS record of members of research cohorts. Instead, OPCS could regularly merge a tape of the cohort members and their identification particulars with OPCS tapes of occurrences of deaths, cancer registrations and/or exits from CHRIS - which would avoid keying in new data, and restrict the computer search to relevant data subsets. This would be appropriate for studies of individuals known to have been alive and resident in England and Wales since 1 January 1991, when

CHRIS was set up, and for studies to evaluate specific screening practices, where the relevant outcomes may be restricted to a limited number of cancers or causes of death.

OPCS is also launching other new services: a facility known as 'list cleaning', introduced in 1994, enables providers in the health service to update information about their patients' vital statistics and residence. In 1995, the CHRIS database will also play a key role when new NHS numbers are issued.

Confidentiality and ethical constraints

Any application to use OPCS' medical research services is examined by the Chief Medical Statistician. He looks for evidence that the applicant is a genuine researcher, and that the work is to advance medical knowledge. The description of the research will then be examined to ensure that the study meets OPCS ethical and confidentiality criteria. For questions involving particular medical aspects, for example the release of individual named cancer registration data, or when the researcher wishes to make personal contact with study members or their families, OPCS would seek independent advice.

Some studies require access to patients' medical records and/or the patients themselves, and here we work within the guidelines of DH's advice on Local Research Ethics Committees (LREC)[11]. These guidelines are clear that researchers must consult an LREC about any research proposal involving access to the medical records of past or present NHS patients. It recognises that epidemiological research through studies of medical records can be extremely valuable, but notes that patients are entitled to regard their medical records as confidential to the NHS, and should in principle be asked if they consent to their own records being released to research workers. OPCS acknowledges that there will be occasions when a researcher will find it difficult or impossible to obtain such consent from every individual, and the LREC will need to be satisfied that the value of such a project outweighs, in the public interest, the principle that individual consent should be obtained. The LREC will also need to be assured that the research will be conducted in accordance with current codes of practice and data protection legislation. Once information has been obtained from the records, no approach shall be made to the patient concerned without the agreement of the health professional currently responsible for their care.

OPCS asks those wanting to use its medical research services to provide evidence that approval has been obtained for their study from an LREC. We also ask to see any planned letter to the FHSAs and to the GPs arrived at after consultation with the LREC. For studies involving possible occupational risk we also ask that the agreement of the workforce has been obtained and that the results are communicated to them or to their representatives. OPCS takes very seriously its responsibility to ensure that any approach to those traced via its facilities is ethical, and does not infringe the constraints of confidentiality. OPCS has clear statements of its values which emphasise its commitments to suppliers of data, the public and its staff as well as to customers - in particular it has published its policies on

confidentiality and security, with a foreword from the Data Protection Registrar[12].

Individual studies must not impinge on these values. The perceived (and legal) risks which may harm OPCS's reputation are considered, as well as the risks of harm to patients or people studied. These must be weighed against benefits to OPCS and to public health and patient care. In the final analysis, OPCS must always be seen to have behaved appropriately as a custodian of the data it holds.

How to get help

To apply to use OPCS services for medical research, an application form (which can be obtained from the Medical Research Section in St Catherine's House) should be completed and returned. OPCS is a non-profit making body, but aims to recover the costs of its contribution to individual studies; any charges depend on whether an automatic computer match can be made and the level of clerical intervention required. Charges are made on a per-case basis, and in 1995/96 charges for flagging range from £0.65 per case for automatic matches to £5.25 per case for difficult-to-trace cases. A small pilot exercise on a sample of data can be done to determine total costs for a given study.

OPCS tries to keep customers (existing and potential) informed about new services which are available, changes in existing services, and changes to charges through its newsletter *The Researcher*, open days at NHSCR in Southport, and by meeting potential customers to discuss proposed studies.

References

1 Snow J. *On the mode of communication of cholera*. London: John Churchill, 1849.

2 *Eighth Report of the Registrar General*. London: General Register Office, 1845.

3 Case RAM and Hosker ME. Tumours of the urinary bladder as an occupational disease in the rubber industry in England and Wales. *Br J Prev Soc Med* , 1954; **8**: 39-50.

4 Doll R and Hill AB. Smoking and cancer. *BMJ*, 1954; **2**:240-1.

5 Baverstock KF, Papworth D and Vennart J. Risks of radiation at low dose rates. *Lancet*, 1981;**1**: 430-3.

6 Newhouse ML and Williams JM. Techniques for tracing past employees: an example from an asbestos factory. *Br J Prev Soc Med*, 1967;**21**:35-9.

7 Greenberg M. Ad hoc occupational mortality studies. In: Drever F, ed. *Occupational health: decennial supplement: the Registrar General's decennial supplement for England and Wales*. London: HMSO, 1995; 235-70. (Series DS; No.10).

8 Office of Population Censuses and Surveys. *Uses of OPCS records for medical research. A review by a Working Group of the Registrar General's Medical Advisory Committee*. London: HMSO, 1993. (OPCS Occasional Paper 41).

9 Stiller CA and Draper GJ. Treatment centre size, entry to trials, and survival in acute lymphoblastic leukaemia. *Arch Dis Child*, 1989; **64**: 657-61.

10 Hedley A J, McMaster W. Use of the National Health Service Central Register for Medical Research Purposes. *Health Bulletin* , 1988; **46**:.63-8.

11 Department of Health. *Local Research Ethics Committees*. Department of Health, 1991.

12 Office of Population Censuses and Surveys. *Statement of policies on confidentiality and security of personal data*. London: OPCS, 1993.

Articles

The demand for primary dental care at a dental teaching hospital, 1989 and 1993

David Thomas*, PhD, Lecturer, **Elias Absi,** PhD, Senior Lecturer, and **Jonathan Shepherd,** PhD, Professor, Department of Oral Surgery, Medicine and Pathology, University of Wales College of Medicine, Heath Park Cardiff CF4 4XY.

Key words: Dental emergency; time trends; contracting.

Health Trends 1995; **27**: 8-11

Summary

The demand for, and provision of, primary dental care was investigated in a teaching hospital setting in 1989 and 1993 - a period which saw the introduction of the new dental contract and the publication of the Poswillo report on general anaesthesia and sedation. Five hundred patients who attended the primary care department for the first time at the University of Wales Dental Hospital were interviewed in May/June 1989, and a further 520 patients were interviewed in May/June 1993. Self-referrals increased from 260 patients (52%) in 1989 to 352 patients (68%) in 1993. The proportion of patients who did not have a general dental practitioner (GDP) increased from 32% (160) in 1989 to 39% (202) in 1993. More patients registered with a dentist self-referred in 1993 compared to those in 1989, reportedly because of inability to obtain an appointment with their own GDP (88), rather than because of cost (17). Over the four-year period there was an increase in demand for treatment of early stage (pulpitic) dental infection from 32% to 40%, and a decrease in relation to end-stage infection (dentoalveolar abscess) from 11% to 6%. This 'safety net' role of dental hospitals needs to be taken into account when contracting for services.

Introduction

Since 1989, the provision of dental services in the United Kingdom (UK) has undergone fundamental changes including the introduction of the new dental contract, with an increasing proportion of the cost of treatment being borne by patients[1], and the implementation of the Poswillo Report on general anaesthesia and sedation in dentistry[2]. A previous national audit demonstrated changes in both general dental service (GDS) and hospital practice of oral surgery in England and Wales[3], indicating decreases in the number of patients waiting for inpatient treatment, increased day-patient throughput, and increasing numbers of minor oral surgical procedures carried out in the GDS. It is not clear, however, whether these changes have been reflected in alterations in the referral pattern and treatment of patients in dental teaching hospital examination and emergency departments. This study compared data obtained at the University of Wales Dental Hospital in 1989 and 1993, a period in which the throughput of patients in the examination and emergency department increased by 26.6%.

*Correspondent: Dr D Thomas

Method

Five hundred consecutive new patients attending the examination and emergency department of the Cardiff Dental Hospital for the first time were interviewed in the months of May and June in 1989, and the exercise was repeated over the same number of days in 1993 (n = 520 patients) - no patients were included in both groups. Patients were asked to indicate their most important reason for self-referral; the remaining portion of the form which categorised their complaints and treatment received, was completed by the examining clinician. To investigate changes in oral surgery treatment, individuals subsequently seen in the oral surgery department for consultation, non-interventive and surgical treatment were investigated as a sub-group. Oral surgery services include provision of more extensive surgical treatment such as extraction of teeth under general anaesthesia (GA). These data were analysed by use of the Pearson statistical Chi-squared test.

Results

There were 1,020 patients in the study (mean age 38.75, range 15-94; SD 16.75), of whom 357 (35%) lived over 10 miles from the hospital (there was no difference between the two study years in relation to this distance). The referral patterns of patients were significantly different in 1989 and 1993 (p <0.01). The proportion of self-referred patients increased from 52% (260) in 1989 to 68% (352) in 1993, and the proportion referred by GDPs fell from 38% (190) to 24% (124) (see Figure 1). The patients' reasons for self-referral were significantly different in 1989 and 1993 (p <0.001) (see Figure 2). The proportion of patients who did not have a GDP rose from 32% (160) in 1989 to 39% (202); in 1993. The proportion of patients without a GDP who were self-referred decreased from 61% (159) in 1989 to 44% (153) in 1993.

Significant changes (p<0.01) were also evident in relation to presenting complaints (see Figure 3). The proportion of patients presenting with pulpal pain increased from 32% (160) in 1989 to 46% (239) in 1993. The proportion of patients with problems requiring oral-surgery (extractions, drainage of abscesses, temporomandibular joint [TMJ] related problems) decreased from 28% (140) in 1989 to 15% (78) in 1993. The number of complaints about dentures decreased from 7.5% (38) in 1989 to 4% (21) in 1993. The treatment provided showed changes between 1989 and 1993 (p < 0.01) (see Figure 4), including an increase in the proportion of patients receiving no active treatment. Decreases were evident in the proportion of denture

Figure 1: *Sources of referral to dental hospital primary care unit, 1989 and 1993*

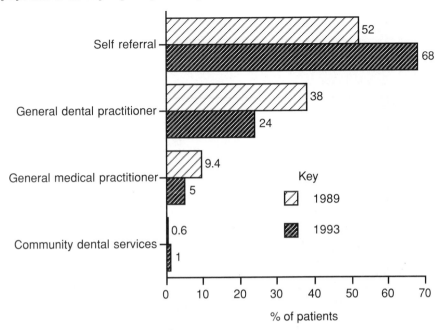

problems and fractured teeth, and the proportion for whom extraction under GA was prescribed. However, there was an increase in the proportion of patients for whom extractions were performed under local anaesthesia (LA), from 29% (146) in 1989 to 36% (185) in 1993.

Oral surgery patients
The patients treated in the oral surgery department in 1993 (227) were of similar age (mean 37.79; range 17-94; SD 15.84) and sex (1.1 male : 1 female) as other patients, but only 52% (118) were registered with a GDP compared with the overall study population of 61% (317); 73% (166) of the patients in this sub-group were self-referred (68 % overall). The presenting complaints in this group were similar to those seen in the overall study population. Pulpal (70%; 159) and periodontal (15%; 34) symptoms and pericoronitis (11%; 25) were more frequent than either trauma (2.3%; 5) or jaw joint (1.2%; 3) complaints.

Overall, the proportion of patients for whom extractions were

performed relative to other treatments did not change: 35% (175) patients in 1989; 36.5% (190) in 1993, although the method of anaesthesia changed substantially. The proportion of patients for whom extractions were performed under LA increased markedly from 63% in 1989 to 82% patients in 1993. The treatment prescribed for patients seen in the oral surgery department in the two study years was significantly different (p <0.001). The proportion of patients for whom extractions were carried out under GA fell from 11% (25) to 0.5% (3) (see Figure 5), as did the proportion for whom incision and drainage of abcesses was carried out 11%, (25) to 6% (13). The proportions of non-surgical treatments for the relief of pain (such as topical medication for pericoronitis and psychotherapy for TMJ dysfunction) did not change (11% of cases for both years).

Discussion
The patterns of referral for, and provision of, emergency treatment at the only dental hospital examination and emergency

Figure 2: *Reasons for referral to the primary care unit, 1989 and 1993*

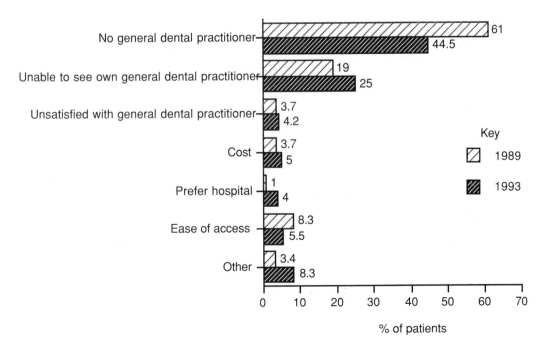

Figure 3: *Presenting complaints of new patients attending the primary care unit, 1989 and 1993*

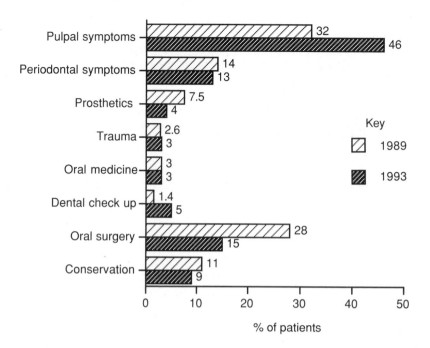

department in Wales underwent substantial changes between 1989 and 1993. Whilst the demographic characteristics of the populations appeared not to change (age, sex and distance from residence to hospital), substantial and clinically significant changes in patient throughput (a 26% increase), referral pattern and treatment were evident.

The decrease in the number of patients referred to the examination and emergency department by GDPs and general medical practitioners may reflect increased registration and commitment to continuous dental care, increased confidence and number of new dental graduates[4], or greater use of direct routes of referral for specialist treatment. The substantial rise in the number of new patient attendances, together with the marked increase in the number of self-referrals, demonstrates an overall increased utilisation of primary care services. There is also a

sizeable minority of patients not registered in the GDS who are inappropriately turning to the hospital service for care.

Reasons for the increase in the numbers of self-referrals are unclear. Despite a marked decrease in the number of self-referred patients who did not have a GDP there was an increase in the number of registered patients claiming to be unable to see a GDP. Dental practitioners are, however, contractually obliged to see their own National Health Service (NHS) patients for emergency treatment within a reasonable period of time[1]. It is unlikely that NHS treatment was inaccessible to these patients; the Family Health Services Authority (FHSA) registered GDP to patient ratio in South Glamorgan fell from 3,636:1 in 1989 to 2,919:1 in 1993. This apparent anomaly may reflect the fact that treatment at the dental hospital is free at the point of delivery, although less than 5% of patients cited cost as a reason for self-

Figure 4: *Treatment provided for new patients attending the primary care unit, 1989 and 1993*

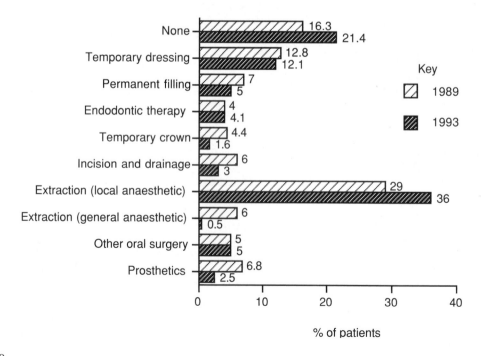

Figure 5: *Treatment administered in the oral surgery department to patients referred from primary care, 1989 and 1993*

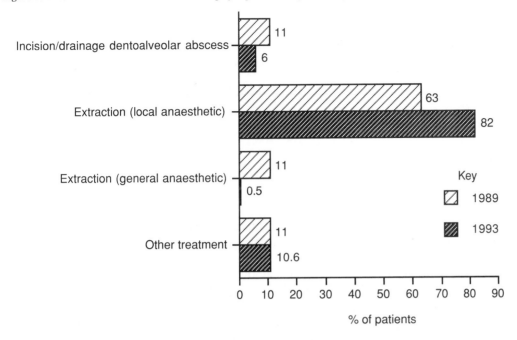

% of patients

referral. A disturbing finding for the dental services as a whole is that over 30% of the patients in this study (and 48% of the patients referred to the oral surgery unit) were not registered with a GDP, and therefore outside any health screening programme instigated in the GDS[5].

In relation to presenting complaints, numbers of patients with pulpal pain, the commonest complaint in other studies[6], increased over the four years, and this occurred with decreases in the numbers of patients presenting with oral surgery complaints (see Figure 3). The relatively low numbers of patients with dento-alveolar trauma in both years may reflect the direct routes of referral to child dental health, or oral surgery departments via accident and emergency departments. It was found that, despite decreases in the caries rate over the same period[7], extraction of teeth under LA was the most commonly performed surgical treatment in both 1989 and 1993. Referral rates for restorative treatment did not change.

Oral surgery patients were found to be of a similar age and lived a similar distance from the hospital as other patients. The principal complaint of oral surgery patients was related to pulpal pain (63%), although 73% of the patients were self-referred and could have been treated in the GDS. The treatment pattern was different in 1993 compared to 1989, particularly in respect of lower numbers of extractions performed under GA and higher numbers of extractions carried out under LA in 1993. These figures reflect policy changes on the part of emergency dental staff to avoid extractions under GA wherever possible, and the increasing use of LA with intravenous sedation as a suitable and economic alternative in anxious patients[3]. Decreases in the number of abcesses drained may reflect the more widespread recognition and early treatment of caries in the primary care setting by both GDPs, and general medical practitioners, particularly in the context of increased registration in the GDS. This suggests that people may recognise the need for dental treatment at an earlier stage now than in the past, wherever they seek treatment.

Conclusion

Despite the encouragement of universal patient registration and primary care in the GDS, the primary care workload of this teaching hospital rose substantially, with associated cost and manpower implications (an increase of three practitioner sessions per week; the appointment of a further full-time dental nurse, and a 30% increase in the cost of consumables). Changes have occurred in the characteristics of patients utilising this service, which may reflect changes in the structure of the GDS - a substantial number of patients who could be treated in the GDS are self-referred and there are large numbers of people, (mostly unregistered), for whom extraction is the treatment of choice. Account should be taken of the 'safety net' role of dental hospitals when contracting for services with these provider units.

Acknowledgement

We thank Professor Norman Whitehouse for his advice on the preparation of this manuscript.

References

1   Department of Health. *General Dental Services (Miscellaneous Amendments) Regulations 1990*. London: HMSO, 1990. (Statutory Instrument 1990: No. 163).

2   Department of Health. *General anaesthesia, sedation and resuscitation in dentistry: report of an Expert Working Party: clinical recommendations.* London: Department of Health, 1991.

3   Thomas DW, Smith, AT, Walker R, Shepherd JP. Provision of Oral and Maxillofacial Surgery services in England & Wales 1984-1991. *Br Dent J* 1994; **176**: 215-9.

4   Matthews RW, Porter SR, Scully C, Levers BGH. Confidence levels of new UK dental graduates. *J Dent Res* 1991; **70**: 726.

5   Zakrzewska JM, Hindle I, Speight PM. Practical considerations for the establishment of an oral cancer screening programme. *Community Dent Health* 1993;**10(suppl 1)**:79-85.

6   Matthews RW, Scully C, Porter K, Griffiths M. An analysis of conditions presenting to a dental hospital emergency clinic. *Health Trends* 1992; **24**: 126-8.

7   Winter G B. Epidemiology of dental caries. *Arch Oral Biol* 1990; **35:** 1s-7s.

Dentists' responses to drug misusers

Mary Dawkes, BA (Hons), GP Liaison Worker, **Sarah Sparkes**, RMN, Psychiatric Nurse, **Mike Smith**, BA, Co-ordinator and **Tom Carnwath***, MRCPsych, Consultant Psychiatrist, Community Drug Team, Chapel Road, Sale, Manchester M33 1FD.

Key words: Dentist; substance abuse; infection control.

Health Trends 1995; **27**: 12-4

Summary

A survey among a sample of illicit drug misusers in 1993 indicated under-use of dental services, in spite of a high prevalence of dental problems, whilst a survey of dentists revealed reluctance to treat such patients. Most dentists use additional infection control procedures when they detect 'at-risk' patients, but their screening procedures are unlikely to be effective. Most dentists in the survey would welcome extra training focused on drug misuse.

Introduction

Dental problems are common among drug misusers[1], and may reflect poor hygiene and diet; the under-use of dental services; gingival damage caused by cocaine application[2]; the high sugar content of the methadone mixture which is widely prescribed to opiate misusers[3]; and oral manifestations of systemic diseases, including HIV infection. We investigated whether under-use of dental services occurred in Trafford, and whether such use was matched by a similar reluctance by dentists to treat drug misusers. In the anticipation that dentists would be anxious about the spread of infection[4], attention was focused on infection control procedures, and in particular whether dentists were following British Dental Association (BDA) guidelines[5].

These BDA guidelines include the following points: "To minimise the risk of transmission between patients and clinical staff, a sensible and practical routine for the prevention of infection and cross-infection should be followed with every patient...dental clinicians have a general obligation to provide care to those in need, and this should extend to infected patients who should be offered the same high standard of care which is available to any other patient...refusing to treat those patients whose infective status is definitely known is illogical, since undiagnosed carriers of infectious diseases pass through the dental surgery every day...those with HIV who are otherwise well and hepatitis B virus carriers may be treated routinely in general dental practice. HIV-positive patients who show evidence of disease or oral manifestations should be referred for expert advice."

Trafford District Health Authority (DHA) lies to the west of Manchester: it includes prosperous suburbs and deprived inner-city areas. The prevalence of drug misuse is high: about 225 people receive treatment for opiate dependency, but it is estimated that there are over 1,000 people dependent on opiates (0.5% of the total population). Amphetamine and heroin use are well established, and cocaine, ecstasy and lysergic acid diethylamide (LSD) use have increased over recent years. Treatment is provided mostly by the community drug team (CDT), which is also responsible for drug training in the District. Anonymous saliva testing of CDT clients indicates that 35% are hepatitis B carriers, and 1% are HIV positive[6]. HIV infection among intravenous drug misusers varies widely across the country: the figures in Manchester are similar to those in Liverpool, whereas in London the estimate of HIV infection is 10%[7] and in Edinburgh is 31%[8].

Method

A questionnaire was sent out in 1993 to all 90 practising dentists in Trafford DHA, who were invited to complete the questionnaires anonymously. A choice of responses was suggested for most questions, but with space for other comments where appropriate. All dentists received a second letter and a follow-up telephone call, asking them to complete the questionnaire if they had not already done so. At the same time a short questionnaire concerning dental care was also given to 32 CDT clients (the caseload of one key-worker). Since clients are allocated to key-workers on a rotational basis, this was considered a reasonably representative sample of CDT clients. Previous experience led us to anticipate a high-response rate, as CDT clients are used to completing questionnaires as part of their regular health assessments, and response is encouraged by the close working relationship with the key-worker.

Results were analysed using the statistical programme for the social sciences (SPSS) by a computer, and significant associations were determined by use of the Chi-square test.

Results

Drug clinic clients

All 32 selected clients completed the questionnaire, and all gave full responses to open-ended questions, such as "What care do you take of your teeth?". Seventeen (53%) reported current problems with their teeth, and five (16%) did not brush their teeth daily. Twenty-one (66%) were registered with a dentist; nine (28%) had not attended a dentist in the previous two years, 11 (34%) had attended three or less times, and 12 (38%) attended their dentist regularly. Of those who never attended a dentist, six (66%) said it was because they were frightened, and three (33%) put the blame on their lifestyle. Only one client (3%) reported having been asked by a dentist whether they had had an HIV test: four (12%) had been asked about hepatitis B infection.

*Correspondent: Dr T Carnwath

Table 1: *Dentists' history taking concerning drugs, hepatitis B and HIV (n=55)*

	All patients asked	Some patients asked	No patients asked
Prescribed drugs	48	6	1
Illicit drugs	1	12	42
Hepatitis B status	37	8	10
HIV status	9	11	35

Dentists

Fifty-five of the 90 questionnaires sent out were returned completed, a response rate of 61%; 17 (31%) dentists chose to include their names, while 38 (69%) preferred to remain anonymous.

History taking

There were large variations between dentists in their approach to history taking with relation to drugs, hepatitis and HIV infection (see Table 1). Whereas most dentists asked patients about prescribed drugs and hepatitis infection, they tended to be far more selective in asking about HIV infection and drug misuse. Of those dentists who were selective in inquiring about drug misuse, 26 (47%) were prompted to do so by the patients' appearance, and 29 (55%) by their behaviour. Dentists who did not ask about drug misuse, chose to do so for the following reasons: fear of offending the patient - 22 (40%), doubt about receiving an honest answer - 28 (51%), and not part of their routine - 17 (31%).

Table 2 *Dentists' response to patient use of various illicit drugs(n=55)*

	Ask more about drug use	Take extra ICPs[1]	Refuse to treat	Seek expert advice
Ecstasy	32	10	3	22
Cocaine	32	13	4	22
Amphetamine	32	13	3	23
Heroin	34	16	7	22
LSD	29	12	3	24
Cannabis	29	10	3	19
Benzodiazepines	30	11	3	15
Other opiates	35	14	3	23

Note: more than one response was possible to this question
[1] Infection control procedures

Response to disclosure of drug use

Dentists were asked how they would respond if they found that their patients were taking various illicit drugs (see Table 2). There were large differences between dentists in their individual responses, although, surprisingly, there were no significant differences in responses to individual drugs - for example between disclosure of heroin and cannabis misuse. Of those dentists using extra infection control procedures, 40% mentioned treating patients at the end of clinics, and 60% mentioned gloves, double gloves, masks and eye protection. There was no significant association between dentists who asked about drug

misuse, and those who would take extra measures to control infection if it was disclosed. Of those dentists who would seek expert advice, 10 would consult the dental hospital, nine a general medical practitioner (GP) and three the CDT. Several dentists mentioned local services that did not actually exist.

Response to disclosure of infection

There was wide variation between dentists in their response to patients infected with hepatitis B or HIV (see Table 3), and those who refused to treat infected patients did so because they felt it was too great a risk to themselves, their staff and other patients - most of them would refer patients to a dental hospital. A large variety of extra infection control procedures were identified by different dentists as being needed if treatment was undertaken for infected patients (see Table 4). Generally, dentists identified the same list of procedures for both hepatitis B and HIV infection.

Training needs

Fifty-one (92%) had read the BDA guidelines on cross-infection control; 47 (86%) wanted to be offered training and information about treating drug misusers, and patients infected with hepatitis B and HIV; 32 (58%) wanted written information and a training seminar, and 29 (53%) also wanted training for their dental surgery assistants, and leaflets for distribution to patients.

Acceptance of referrals from community drug team

Five (9%) dentists were willing to accept CDT clients referred by staff for dental treatment, and the same five (9%) were willing to accept hepatitis B positive patients, and six (11%) (including the previous five) were willing to accept HIV positive patients.

Discussion

The client survey indicates that dental problems are widespread among drug misusers, and that dental services are poorly used. Only 38% attended their dentist every six months, although 53% reported ongoing problems with their teeth. (The most recent Office of Population Censuses and Surveys [OPCS] survey found that in the general population, 48% of people in this age-group attend for regular dental check-ups[9]). There is also a corresponding reluctance on the part of dentists to treat drug misusers. Only five (9%) were willing to accept referral of patients from the CDT; however, most were willing to treat current patients whom they discovered were drug misusers.

The BDA advocates a 'one-tier' approach to infection control procedures, on the grounds that it is impossible to know which patients are infected. Twenty-nine per cent of dentists surveyed would take extra measures if heroin misuse were disclosed, rising to over 65% for those treating patients with hepatitis B or who were HIV positive. The problem with using such a selective 'two-tier' approach is that it is hard to know who should be selected for extra precautions. It is also possible that at-risk patients might be less likely to be honest if they know that

Table 3: *Response of dentists to patient infection with HIV and Hepatitis B (n=55)*

	Willing to treat	Take extra ICPs[1]	Refuse to treat	Refer elsewhere	Seek advice
Hepatitis B +ve	46	30	9	5	8
HIV+ve asymptomatic	30	31	3	13	11
HIV+ve symptomatic	21	22	6	31	15

Note: more than one response was possible to this question
[1] Infection control procedures

Table 4: *Number of dentists volunteering particular procedures as needed as additional measures when treating patients infected with HIV or hepatitis B (among those willing to offer treatment)*

Procedure	Hepatitis B (n=46)	HIV(n=30)
Book last appointment of day	16	20
Gloves	3	6
Double gloves	2	4
Eye protection	4	7
Face mask	5	8
Separate waste disposal	4	3
Longer sterilisation of instruments	2	3
Autoclave before and after treatment twice	1	1
Disposal of diamond burrs	0	1
Avoidance of high speed drill	3	2
Double check normal procedures	3	2
Separate autoclaving	3	4
Change of clothes	0	1
Protective gowns	3	5
DSA[1] protection	0	4
Sterilise burrs and handpieces	2	4
Cellophane-wrap chair and structures	1	1
Full disinfection procedure	3	5
Cover work surfaces	0	2

Note: more than one response was possible to this question

[1] Dental surgeon's assistant

disclosure would be met with extra infection control procedures, which may be seen as stigmatising.

Even if it is accepted that a two-tier approach is practicable, inconsistencies are revealed by this survey - dentists who believe in taking extra precautions are not necessarily the same ones who ask about drug misuse. Few of the surveyed CDT clients were asked about drug misuse, which is consistent with the dentists' survey, in which only a minority of dentists regularly asked about drug misuse. Presumably, at-risk patients are not detected.

It is of interest that there was no significant difference between the response to different drugs when misuse was detected - 18% of dentists would use extra infection control procedures if they learnt about cannabis use. It has been estimated that 20-30% of people under the age of 30 years have tried cannabis at some time[10], and that only a very small minority of these will be intravenous drug misusers. If cannabis misuse really justified using extra precautions against infection, then the logical response would be to employ them with all people between 15 and 30 years-of-age.

Eighty-five per cent of dentists surveyed requested more training about drug misuse. That this would be desirable is indicated by lack of knowledge concerning local treatment facilities, and inconsistencies in response to disclosure of drug misuse.

Conclusion

Our study indicated a lack of consistency about the treatment by dentists in our sample of drug misusers. The clear demand from the surveyed dentists for more training and information about local treatment facilities should be considered by all purchasers of health care.

Acknowledgements

We thank Dr A Crawford (District Dental Officer, South Manchester), Dr Siobhan Hudson Davies (Senior research officer, Manchester University) and Dr C Quigley (Consultant in Public Health, Trafford Health Authority), for their help in drawing up the questionnaire and for their work in helping to persuade local practitioners to complete it.

References

[1] Scheutz F. Dental health in a group of drug addicts attending an addiction clinic. *Commun Dent Oral Epidemiol* 1984; **12:** 23-38.

[2] Quart AM, Small AB, Klein RS. The cocaine connection: users imperil their gingiva. *J Am Dent Assoc* 1991; **122:** 85-7.

[3] Bigwood CS, Coelho AJ. Methadone and caries. *Br Dent J* 1990; **168:** 231.

[4] Hardie J. Concerns regarding infection control recommendations for dental practice. *J Can Dent Assoc* 1992; **58:** 377-8, 382-6.

[5] British Dental Association Advisory Service. *The control of cross-infection in dentistry*. London: British Dental Association, 1991.

[6] The unlinked anonymous HIV prevalence monitoring programme in England and Wales: preliminary results. *CDR (Lond-Engl-Rev)* 1991; **1:** 69-76.

[7] Stimson G, Quirk A. *Drugs: the state of the region: a profile of drug and alcohol problems in North West Thames Regional Health Authority*. London: The Centre for Research on Drugs and Health Behaviour, 1992.

[8] Ronald PJ, Robertson JR. Prevalence of HIV infection among drug users in Edinburgh. *BMJ* 1992; **304:** 1506.

[9] Todd TE, Lader D. *Adult dental health: United Kingdom: 1988*. London: HMSO, 1991.

[10] Gallup Surveys. *The youth report*. London: Gallup/Wrangler, 1992.

Maternity services for drug misusers in England and Wales: a national survey

Clive Morrison*, MB ChB, Senior Clinical Medical Officer for Special Groups and Obstetric Liaison Officer in Drug Dependency, The Maryland Centre, 8 Maryland Street, Liverpool L1 9DE and **Catherine Siney**, SRN, Drugs Liaison Midwife, Liverpool Women's Hospital, Crown Street, Liverpool, L8 7SS.

Keywords: Drug misuse; obstetric liaison; drug use in pregnancy; neonatal opiate withdrawal; HIV/HBV.

Health Trends 1995; **27**: 15-7

Summary

A postal questionnaire was sent to the 213 National Health Service maternity units in England and Wales to identify their current involvement with drug misusers. The response rate was 89.5%. Data indicated that only 29% had formal links with their local drug agency. Child protection case conferences were automatically convened in 52%, and 57% routinely admitted babies to high dependency areas. Twenty-seven per cent of the units did not offer hepatitis B screening to pregnant women, and 32% did not offer hepatitis B prophylaxis to babies whose mothers were infected.

Local Health purchasing authorities should ensure that their providers are offering appropriate services to pregnant drug misusers in order to encourage such women to seek help without fear of discrimination. Liaison between health care agencies should be encouraged and areas with low levels of drug misuse should receive help with formulating policies, and training, from units with more experience.

Introduction

The 1989 report of the Advisory Council on the Misuse of Drugs (ACMD)[1] recognised that maternity services would experience an increase in the number of pregnant women who are misusing drugs. It advised that in areas which have a high prevalence of drug misuse, maternity staff should be trained in managing pregnancies in drug misusers, and that there should be good two-way referral between obstetric and specialist drug services. In response, differing models of care have been provided throughout the United Kingdom[2,3,4].

During the six months to 31 March 1993, 3,964 females of child-bearing age (15-39 years old) presented with a drug misuse problem (22% of all misusers) as recorded by Regional Drug Misuse Databases[5]. For all individuals misusing drugs, 91% misused heroin, methadone or other opiates, 35% misused stimulant drugs such as cocaine and amphetamines, and various other substances such as cannabis (25%), benzodiazepines (22%), and hallucinogens (7%) were also misused. At least 25% misused more than one drug, and 38% currently injected their main drug. We surveyed 213 maternity units in England and Wales to quantify drug misuse in pregnancy, and how well maternity services have responded to the ACMD report.

* Correspondent: Dr C Morrison

Method

In February 1993, a postal questionnaire was sent to the clinical directors of 213 obstetric and maternity units about contact with pregnant female drug misusers, (as classified under the Misuse of Drugs Act 1971). Telephone and postal reminders were sent to non-responders.

The questionnaire asked for information on: the number of births in drug misusing mothers each year; how these women were managed by the possibility of referral; what type of agency was available; and what type of drug treatment was offered. Information on policies for HIV and hepatitis B screening and treatment was also requested, as were details on the extent of social service involvement and intervention to drug misusing mothers regarding child protection case conferences.

Results

A total of 191 units (89.5%) responded, reporting a total of 568 births annually to drug misusing women (Table 1). There was a wide variation in the number of units involved in the care of pregnant drug misusers in each region and overall, units in the North Thames Regional Health Authorities (RHA) had the most experience: 27 units that responded to our questionnaire (of 33) indicated that 24 centres had delivered babies to drug misusing women. The estimated number of deliveries in the previous 12 months varied from 8 to 167: Mersey RHA had a rate of deliveries to drug misusing women per 10,000 total deliveries which was two and a half times greater than the second highest region, the North Western RHA.

Fifty-seven maternity units (29.8%) had formal referral policies to drug agencies for pregnant women identified as drug misusers. Forty-two units (22%) had access to local health authority National Health Service (NHS) drug dependency clinics, 48 (25.1%) to community drug teams and 17 (8.9%) to voluntary and non-statutory agencies. Seventy-four units (38.7%) had access to agencies that were able to prescribe methadone. Four units reported that general practitioners (GPs) were prepared to offer drug dependency treatment in their care of pregnant addicts.

Over half of the units (100 [52.4%]) automatically convened child protection case conferences on all babies born to drug misusing mothers, and 109 units (57.1%) had policies in which newborn babies were automatically separated at birth from their mothers to be admitted to a special care baby unit, or neonatal intensive care unit for observation or treatment.

Table 1: *Incidence of deliveries to drug-misusing women by total number of deliveries and notification of female addicts*

Region	No. of units	Response rate (%)	% of Units with drug-misusing mothers delivering in last 12 months	Estimated no of deliveries to drug-misusing mothers in in previous 12 months	Rate per 10000 deliveries[1]	Rate per notification of 1000 female addicts[2]
Northern	19	84.2	50.0	8	1.9	190.5
Yorkshire	19	84.2	37.5	11	2.2	65.5
Trent	11	100	27.3	10	1.6	80.6
East Anglia	8	100	37.5	11	4.2	68.3
North West Thames [3]	17	82.3	92.9	66	12.8	108.6
North East Thames	16	81.3	84.6	41	7.2	47.7
South East Thames	18	88.9	68.7	61	11.7	137.4
South West Thames	13	100	69.2	25	6.3	77.6
Wessex	10	100	50.0	11	3.0	75.9
Oxford	9	100	44.4	14	3.8	115.7
South Western	11	100	27.3	6	1.5	25.0
West Midlands	20	95.0	47.4	12	1.6	50.0
Mersey	9	88.9	87.5	167	50.1	166.0
North Western	17	76.5	61.5	106	18.7	179.1
Wales	16	87.5	64.3	19	4.9	91.3
Total	213	89.7	57.1	568	8.1	111.9

[1] Office of Population Censuses and Surveys Birth Statistics 1991. England and Wales. HMSO London.
[2] Home Office data from the Addicts Index January to December 1991.
[3] Including Special Health Authority.

Forty-five units (23.6%) universally screened for hepatitis B and 94 (49.2%) selectively screened drug misusers. Only 129 (67.5%) had policies to offer hepatitis B immunoglobulin and vaccination to babies of mothers who are carriers of hepatitis B (HBsAg positive).

Seventy-five (39.3%) units routinely offered HIV tests to drug misusers, and 8 (4.2%) automatically tested. Pre-test HIV counselling was undertaken by consultant obstetricians in 64 (33.5%) units, by general midwifery staff in 17 units (8.9%) and by junior medical staff in 5 units (2.6%). Twenty-four units (12.6%) had designated counsellor midwives and in 69 units (36.1%) HIV counselling was performed by outside agencies such as genito-urinary medicine clinics. GPs, HIV counsellors in local AIDS units, social workers, HIV specialist and infection control nurses, or keyworkers from drug agencies. Of the 134 units who had performed an HIV test in the last 12 months, only 51.5% (69/134) had counsellors who had attended HIV training courses or had qualifications in counselling.

Discussion

Over the 12 months prior to the completion of the survey there were approximately 568 babies born to women drug misusers in England and Wales. Although some Regions experience higher rates of drug misuse than others, all maternity units should be capable of identifying pregnant misusers. However, it appears that those units with more experience of seeing pregnant drug misusers are more adept at identifying such women. Nationally, over 11% of the total number of female drug misusers notified have given birth. Generally, Regions with the highest prevalence also recognised a greater proportion of pregnant drug misusers. The exception in this study was North East Thames Region which notified the second largest number of drug misusers, but

identified less than half the national average of pregnancies per 1,000 female drug misusers. Although this rate should be viewed with caution due to differences in the notification of drug misusers and in fertility rates between Regions, it does indicate that some Regions may need to examine why they have low recognition of pregnant drug misusers, and whether appropriate services are being offered to those who are identified.

Less than a third of units had a liaison service and formal referral policies when pregnant drug misusers were identified in antenatal clinics. Less than half of units referred to drug agencies that prescribed methadone, despite the advantages of such treatment programmes[6].

The Department of Health (DH) has been encouraging GPs to become more involved in the care of drug misusers in primary care. However, only a small number of units reported that GPs were prepared to take an active role in the management of the drug problem, although they would continue to participate in shared antenatal care. This may reflect a preference to refer such patients to specialist services.

In an attempt to avoid statutory services, possibly due to a fear of their children being taken into social services care, women drug misusers often present late to services when pregnant. The ACMD advised[7] that such mothers should not be deterred from seeking help and that social services departments should ensure that drug misuse alone is never perceived or used as a reason for separating parent and child. Despite this, a majority of units still automatically convene child protection case conferences - often entailing detention of the baby in hospital for several days after the mother has been discharged, until the conference has decided upon the level of further social services involvement. Another way misusers are stigmatised is by the immediate separation of babies from the mother at birth to be monitored in intensive care units. This occurred in over half the units surveyed, and could cause problems in mother-child bonding. Experienced units describe low rates of neonatal withdrawal[4] and most cases were easily managed on post-natal wards without the need for separation.

A quarter of units universally screen for hepatitis B, and a further 49% selectively test drug users. Reports have suggested that universal screening programmes are more efficient than selective programmes at identifying current hepatitis B infection[8]. More than a quarter of the units did not offer hepatitis B screening, whilst nearly a third did not offer treatment to prevent the mother to baby transfer of hepatitis B infection - despite guidelines reporting the benefits of prophylaxis[9,10,11].

The DH has recommended that maternity units offer voluntary named HIV testing at antenatal clinics in areas of high HIV seroprevalence[12]. More provincial antenatal clinics (45% [57/127]), offered HIV testing than clinics in the Thames Regions (40% [26/64]), and testing is probably only cost effective in the London Regions, as HIV prevalence remains low elsewhere[13] and can cost up to £181,000 per HIV-positive result[14]. Selectively offering HIV tests to drug misusers can be seen as stigmatising, especially to women who have never injected drugs.

Eight units automatically tested drug misusers for HIV infection despite DH guidelines, and contrary to General Medical Council ethical guidance, (testing for HIV antibodies should only be performed with the woman's explicit consent). Pre-test discussion and information should be provided by a midwife or doctor who has received education and training about HIV, but only half the units reported that they had such trained staff[15]. A minority of units (12.6%) had a counsellor midwife and over a third relied upon outside agencies for support as they felt there was insufficient training of midwifery staff for them to have the necessary counselling skills[16]. It has been recommended that in areas where the probability of infection is low, it is unreasonable to conduct intensive counselling, but there should be written material available[17]. However, the uptake of HIV testing remains low even in centres that encourage HIV testing[18].

Conclusion

There appears to be a wide variation between Regions in the recognition of pregnant drug misusers, and a significant proportion of maternity units continue with policies that stigmatise and marginalise drug misusers. Local health purchasers should undertake needs assessment to ensure that services are appropriate and encourage healthy alliances and liaisons between maternity services and drug agencies.

Acknowledgements
We thank all those who returned questionnaires and Ms Evelyn Watson for secretarial support.

References

1 Advisory Council on the Misuse of Drugs. *AIDS and drug misuse: part 2,* . London: HMSO, 1988.

2 Hepburn M. Drug use in pregnancy. *Br J Hosp Med* 1993;**49:** 51-5.

3 Dawe S, Gerada C, Strang J. Establishment of a liaison service for pregnant opiate-dependent women. *Br J Addict* 1992; **87:** 867-71.

4 Morrison CL, Siney C, Ruben SM, Worthington M. Obstetric liaison in drug dependency. *Addiction Research.* In Press

5 Government Statistical Service Drug Misuse Statistics. *Statistical Bulletin* March 1994; London: Department of Health 1994.

6 Ruben S. The implications for drug dependency units. In: Henderson S, ed. *Women, HIV, drugs: practical issues..* London: ISDD, 1990; 52-7.

7 Advisory Council on the Misuse of Drugs. *AIDS and drug misuse: part 1.* London: HMSO, 1988.

8 Chrystie I, Sumner D, Palmer S, Kenny A, Banatvala J. Screening of pregnant women for evidence of current hepatitis B infection: selective or universal? *Health Trends,* 1992; **24:** 13-5.

9 British Paediatric Association. *Manual on infections and immunisations in children* . Oxford: Oxford University Press, 1991.

10 Polakoff S, Vandervelde EM. Immunisation of neonates at high risk of hepatitis B in England and Wales: national surveillance. *BMJ* 1988; **297:** 249-53.

11 Neal KR, Radford JML. Immunisation of children born to mothers positive for anti-HBe. *BMJ* 1992; **304:** 1441.

12 Department of Health. *Additional sites for HIV antibody testing; offering voluntary named HIV antibody testing to women receiving antenatal care; partner notification for HIV infection.* Heywood (Lancashire): Department of Health, 1992. (PL/CO(92) 5).

13 Davison C. National Study of HIV in pregnancy. *Quarterly Newsletter* Issue 17, 1993: AIDS Education and research trust: Horsham.

14 Department of Health. *HIV/AIDS and sexual health.* Heywood (Lancashire): Department of Health, 1993. (Health of the nation key area handbooks).

15 Meadows J, Chester T, Catalán J. Screening for HIV in pregnancy. *BMJ* 1994; **308:** 414-5.

16 Meadows J, Chester T, Catalán J, Sherr L, Stone Y, Gazzard B. Testing for HIV in the antenatal clinic: the views of the midwives. *AIDS Care* 1993: **4:** 157-64.

17 Goldberg DJ, Johnstone FD. Universal named testing of pregnant women for HIV. *BMJ* 1993; **306:** 1144-5.

18 Meadows J, Jenkinson S, Catalán J. Who chooses to have the HIV antibody test in the antenatal clinic? *Midwifery* 1994: **10:** 44-8.

General hospital services for attempted suicide patients: a survey in one Region

Keith Hawton[*], DM, Consultant Pyschiatrist and Senior Clinical Lecturer, University Department of Psychiatry, Warneford Hospital, Oxford OX3 7JX, and **Rachel James**, BA(QTS), Senior Clinical Audit Assistant, Four Counties Clinical Audit Team, Anglia and Oxford Regional Health Authority, Old Road, Headington, Oxford OX3 7LF.

Keywords: Attempted suicide patients; general hospitals; psychiatric services; medical and nursing services; monitoring; guidelines.

Health Trends 1995; **27**: 18-21

Summary

A survey of the general hospital services for attempted suicide patients in one Region indicated that most hospitals fell short of many of the standards contained in the Department of Health 1984 guidelines and the recently established Royal College of Psychiatrists guidelines, particularly with regard to active planning and monitoring of the service, involvement of non-medical clinical staff, availability of the service and the training of staff.

Introduction

Attempted suicide (or deliberate self-harm) is a major health care problem in the United Kingdom (UK), with a conservative estimate of 100,000 general hospital referrals per year[1], nearly 20,000 of these among teenagers[2]. Self-poisoning represents the most common reason for acute medical admission of females to general hospitals and the second most common reason (after ischaemic heart disease) for men[3].

Attempted suicide indicates considerable emotional distress (and often actual psychiatric disorder), and it is also commonly repeated - some 12-20% making a repeat attempt within a year[1,4,5]. It is also often followed by suicide; at least 1% of attempters successfully commit suicide within a year, and some 3% or more during the 3-8 years after a first attempt[6-8].

Clearly there should be an adequate service for suicide attempters in every general hospital. This is of particular relevance to efforts to achieve the suicide targets in *The Health of the Nation*[9]. According to the Department of Health and Social Security (DHSS) 1984 official guidelines, *The management of deliberate self-harm*[10], all attempted suicide patients referred to hospital should receive a psychological assessment by a member of staff specifically trained for this task; there are other recommendations for general hospital care of these patients. Unfortunately, it appears that in some hospitals such services are inadequate; for example, the service may be poorly staffed, not readily available (especially at night and weekends) and lack any means of providing information on the caseload. An unacceptable number of patients may leave hospital without a full assessment[11,12].

[*]Correspondent: Dr K Hawton

To address this problem the Liaison Psychiatry Group of the Royal College of Psychiatrists (RCPsych) held a one-day meeting in November 1992 to establish the consensus guidelines *The General Hospital Management of Adult Self-Harm: A Consensus Statement on Standards for Service Provision*[13]. These guidelines, endorsed by the RCPsych, focus on management of these patients in accident and emergency (A&E) and inpatient general hospital settings, as well as care by psychiatric and non-psychiatric staff, and are designed with ease of audit in mind.

We surveyed general hospitals in the former Oxford Region to identify the nature of the services available for attempted suicide patients, and to assess the adequacy of the services.

Method

The survey included the nine major general hospitals in the former Oxford Region; seven district general hospitals, one teaching hospital and one acute general hospital, ranging in size from 275 to 900 beds, with catchment area populations from approximately 178,000 to approximately 500,000; most hospitals served both rural and urban areas. The overall numbers of new A&E department attendances at individual hospitals during the year 1 April 1991- 31 March 1992 ranged from approximately 18,500 to 65,300.

The questionnaire used for the survey was designed to assess various factors related to attempted suicide patients: the nature of the hospital psychiatric service; the actual or estimated number of suicide attempts referred per year; the age breakdown of the attempters according to sex; the proportion of patients admitted to a hospital bed; whether or not any means was available for monitoring attempted suicide referrals to the hospital; the nature of any audits which were carried out; and whether any protocols and/or training were available to assist staff in the A&E department and in general medical wards in managing these patients. The questionnaire also inquired about any specific service in the general hospital for the psychosocial assessment and aftercare of attempted suicide patients, including: whether a service was available; the nature of any referral policy (including written guidelines); the staffing of the service; its availability and response time (particularly at night and the weekend); whether special arrangements were available for young attempters (under 18 years-of-age) and older attempters (over 60 years-of-age); the availability of specific rooms for conducting interviews with patients and relatives in the A&E department and in medical inpatients units; and the availability and nature of any aftercare. Inquiry was also made about whether there were any particular local people who took a special clinical and/or research interest in attempted suicide patients. Finally, the respondents were asked if they thought the general hospital service for attempted suicide patients could be improved and, if so, how.

The questionnaires were sent out at the beginning of 1993 to clinicians identified as likely to have the best knowledge in each hospital. In some cases this was a psychiatrist, in others an A&E consultant, and sometimes both.

Results

The response rate was 100%, although a few questions were not answered by some respondents. In only four of the nine hospitals was there a system for regular monitoring of the numbers of suicide attempters being referred to the hospital, and in one of these this only recorded cases referred to the psychiatric service.

Attempted suicide patients

The numbers of attempted suicide patients referred to hospital in 1990 and 1991 (the most recent available records) were known for six of the nine hospitals surveyed, and varied between 231 and 962. In all but one of these six hospitals, the sex ratio showed the majority to be women, and in all six hospitals approximately two-thirds of the patients were under 35 years-of-age - characteristics in keeping with the general pattern in the UK[3,14]. The proportion of attempters reported as being admitted to a hospital bed as opposed to being discharged directly from the A&E department varied markedly between the six hospitals, from 39% to 85%, with one hospital indicating a 'possible' figure of 21%.

Medical services for attempted suicide patients

Only three of the nine hospitals reported that they had special 'short-stay' admission beds, the number of beds ranging from seven to nine. In six hospitals, specific guidelines were available on the immediate medical management of attempted suicide patients in the A&E department. Six hospitals reported that some training in the psychosocial assessment of these patients was provided for A&E staff - two of these included teaching by a consultant psychiatrist. No hospital reported that training was provided for general medical or nursing staff.

Psychiatric services

Five hospitals had a psychiatric department within the hospital, four of these having inpatient beds. Six hospitals reported having some psychiatric service for the general hospital, three of these having a psychiatric unit or department on site - however, only two hospitals had a service with a consultant specifically appointed in liaison psychiatry. Six hospitals had a specific service for attempted suicide patients, and in the three remaining hospitals the assessments of these patients were conducted by on-call psychiatrists, but in addition, in two of these the physicians conducted preliminary assessments before deciding whether or not a psychiatrist needed to be involved. Five hospitals had a specific policy regarding referral for assessment by the psychiatric service, all of these having policy documents on the procedures to be followed. In five hospitals there were written guidelines to assist clinicians in the psychiatric assessments of patients.

Staffing and availability

Staffing for attempted suicide patients varied greatly, and only two hospitals reported non-medical staff (psychiatric nurses and social workers) as members of the service. Four services relied primarily on psychiatrists in training to provide the assessments, with consultant supervision and back-up, while one appeared to rely solely on sessions from a consultant psychiatrist. Four hospitals reported that the service was available all the time, although in at least one of those which included non-medical staff, only medical staff were available at night and weekends. The two other hospitals with a service reported that this was only available on weekdays and during the daytime.

Following a request for an emergency assessment of an attempted suicide patient in the A&E department, the time taken before an assessment could take place was routinely less than an hour in only one hospital. In four hospitals the minimum time was between 1-2 hours, although in one of these it might be more than five hours. The time taken in another hospital was generally 2-4 hours (although it might be longer), and in the final hospital it was generally more than 5 hours before an emergency assessment could occur. For routine requests for assessment of patients admitted as inpatients, a psychiatric assessment generally occurred on the same day when a request was made during the first part of the morning (ie 9-11 am), but in three hospitals this was not generally the case, and in seven hospitals an assessment occurred within 24-hours if a referral was made late in the day, but in one the assessment would be delayed longer than this (no information for one hospital for both these items).

Very young and older patients

In seven hospitals there were special arrangements for the assessment of young suicide attempters (under 18 years-of-age) - in six an assessment by a child/adolescent psychiatrist, and in one, involvement of a social worker or counsellor with a special interest in adolescents. Only one hospital had special arrangements for older suicide attempters (over 60 years-of-age), this being close liaison with the psychogeriatric service, with social worker involvement where necessary.

Interview facilities

All of the hospitals reported having rooms available in the A&E department in which attempted suicide patients could be interviewed, but two hospitals reported that such rooms were not available for patients admitted as inpatients.

Availability of information on patients

Only five hospitals reported that information was available on the proportion of admitted attempted suicide patients who were seen for psychiatric assessment. For three hospitals this was stated as 100%, and was 94% and 74% in the other two. The proportion of non-admitted patients discharged from the A&E department who received an assessment was known in only four hospitals, and this varied between 15% and 90%. Information on how many of these patients discharged themselves before a psychiatric assessment could be conducted was only available in four hospitals.

Aftercare
All hospitals reported that at least some patients could receive aftercare from the person who conducted the initial assessment.

Service planning and research
Only one hospital reported having a local group for planning and overseeing the service for attempted suicide patients, and this group comprised psychiatrists only. In six hospitals, however, there was at least one clinician who took a special interest in the general hospital service for these patients, and in five hospitals there was someone who took a specific research or audit interest. Audits were carried out concerning repetition of suicide attempts in three hospitals, of the care offered to attempters after they left hospital, and suicide following attempted suicide in two hospitals, and of compliance with aftercare in one hospital.

Satisfaction with the service for attempted suicide patients
Eight hospitals answered yes to the question of whether or not it was thought that the service available for the psychiatric and social assessment of attempted suicide patients could be improved. Interestingly, the remaining hospital was the one which reported not having a special service for psychosocial assessment of suicide attempters, lacked any means of monitoring the members of admitted or non-admitted suicide attempters, and had no one who took a special interest in either the provision of a clinical service for these patients or research/audit concerning this problem. The responses from the remaining eight hospitals (see Table 1) indicated that the most frequent concerns were about interview facilities, availability of the service and aftercare. Further spontaneous comments indicated that staff in some hospitals would have liked to have had non-medical as well as medical staff available to conduct assessments.

Discussion
This survey provides an overview of the general hospital services for suicide attempters in one Region. It is difficult to assess the validity of the responses obtained - some of those regarding proportions of patients receiving psychosocial assessment seem to be over-estimated in the light of findings based on specific audits[1]. Responses concerning the nature of the service and

Table 1: *Responses from eight hospitals in wihch it was thought that the general hospital service for attempted suicide patients could be improved*

Improvements required	Number responding positively to each item
Better interview facilities in A & E department	5
Better interview facilities on wards	5
Service should be more readily available	4
Improved provision of aftercare	4
Clearer referral policy needed	3
Better availability of service at nights	3
Better availability of service at weekends	3
Reduced length of stay of patients in medical beds	1

suggestions for improvements, however, are likely to be both valid and reliable.

The DHSS 1984 guidelines[10] on the management of deliberate self-harm recommended that in addition to psychiatrists, suitably trained medical staff could undertake psychosocial assessment of patients, and that other specially trained workers could also be involved in care. The guidelines also emphasised the need for Districts to establish policies for additional pre-qualification and in-service training, especially for all junior medical staff and non-medical personnel likely to be working with attempted suicide patients. The results of this survey indicate that 10 years after the guidelines were sent to all District Health Authorities (DHAs), only modest progress has been made in implementing them. There was little evidence of active planning and monitoring of services (although most hospitals had at least one clinician who took a special interest in the service for these patients), only two hospitals included non-medical staff in the service, and while training in the management of attempted suicide patients was provided for A&E staff in six hospitals, none reported any training of this kind for staff on general medical wards.

The guidelines recently developed by the Liaison Psychiatry Group of the RCPsych include broader and more detailed recommendations[13]. The establishment of a self-harm services planning group in each hospital is emphasised, which might include an A&E consultant, psychiatric consultant, A&E nurse, psychiatric nurse, social worker, general practitioner, a representative of purchasers, a provider manager and information officer. There is considerable emphasis on training and supervision of A&E staff, general medical and nursing staff, and of medical and non-medical personnel. Few, if any, of the hospitals in this survey came near to matching this standard. The discharge of substantial proportions of patients from the A&E departments without at least a basic psychosocial assessment is a great cause for concern.

While the RCPsych document accepts that the establishment of a specialist multidisciplinary clinical team may not be feasible in small hospitals, it nevertheless emphasises that some minimum criteria should always be in place. All A&E departments and inpatient units should have facilities allowing private interview of patients and relatives. These criteria were met in nearly all the hospitals in this survey. Services were available in the majority of hospitals (consisting solely of psychiatric staff in all but two), but three relied on the on-call psychiatric service for assessments of patients. In nearly all the hospitals, a specialist assessment could be provided within the maximum recommended time of 3 hours of a patient's arrival in the A&E department, and within 2-4 hours for non-urgent referrals of admitted patients. In only one hospital, however, could a request for an emergency assessment be provided within the recommended maximum time of one hour. In more than half the hospitals there were written guidelines regarding both the policy for referral to the psychiatric service, and the psychiatric assessment procedure for assessment of self-harm patients. There were special arrangements for the assessment of very young attempters, but in only one hospital was there such an arrangement for elderly attempters.

Most hospitals had an adequate system for monitoring basic information on deliberate self-harm patients, however it is worrying, that less than half could provide any information on how many patients left the A&E department without a psychosocial assessment - which also raises the possibility of a hospital being unable to deal with a complaint adequately should a patient die shortly after leaving the hospital.

Responders in all but one hospital thought that the service could be improved; the remaining hospital seemed to have the least adequate service of all the hospitals. The desired improvements particularly concerned interview facilities availability of the service, aftercare and referral policies - all topics which are emphasised in the RCPsych guidelines[13]. Implementation of the guidelines will clearly have resource implications, although meeting some recommendations will only require tightening up on current practice. General hospital services for attempted suicide patients must be a high priority: the proportion of people who die by suicide each year who will have been referred to hospital after a suicide attempt within the preceding year is approximately one in four - prevention of suicide in even a minority of these cases could contribute substantially to the Government's health strategy target[9] of a 15% reduction in the overall suicide rate.

Conclusion
General hospital services for attempted suicide patients require special attention, need to be carefully planned and monitored, should involve non-medical as well as medical staff and include appropriate training and supervision, should be readily available to patients and should have adequate physical facilities. A multidisciplinary planning group for self-harm services should be established in each general hospital or DHA.

Acknowledgements
The authors thank Oxford Regional Health Authority Accident and Emergency Audit Group members for their support of the project and the late Mr Ray Daniels for his help with the design of the questionnaire. We are grateful for the co-operation of the general hospital clinicians who completed the questionnaires. The survey was conducted while Dr Hawton was in receipt of a grant from the Department of Health.

References
1 Hawton K, Fagg J. Trends in deliberate self-poisoning and self-injury in Oxford, 1976-1990. *BMJ* 1992; **304:** 1409-11.

2 Hawton K, Fagg J. Deliberate self-poisoning and self-injury in adolescents: a study of characteristics and trends in Oxford, 1976-89. *Br J Psychiatry* 1992; **161:** 816-23.

3 Hawton K, Catalan J. *Attempted Suicide.* Oxford: Oxford University Press, 1987.

4 Morgan HG, Barton J, Pottle S, Pocock H, Burns-Cox CJ. Deliberate self-harm: a follow-up study of 279 patients. *Br J Psychiatry* 1976; **128:** 361-8.

5 Bancroft J, Marsack P. The repetitiveness of self-poisoning and self-injury. *Br J Psychiatry* 1977; **131:** 394-9.

6 Buglass D, Horton J. A scale for predicting subsequent suicidal behaviour. *Br J Psychiatry* 1974; **124:** 573-8.

7 Hawton K, Fagg J. Suicide and other causes of death following attempted suicide. *Br J Psychiatry* 1988; **152:** 359-66.

8 Nordentoft M, Breum L, Munck LK, Nordestgaard AG, Hunding A, Lawson-Bjaeldager PA. High mortality by natural and unnatural causes: a 10 year follow-up study of patients admitted to a poisoning treatment centre after suicide attempts. *BMJ* 1993; **306:** 1637-41.

9 Department of Health. *The health of the nation: a strategy for health in England.* London: HMSO, 1992. (CM 1986).

10 Department of Health and Social Security. *The management of deliberate self-harm.* Heywood (Lancashire): Department of Health and Social Security, 1984. (Health Notice: HN(84)25).

11 Owens DW, Jones SJ. The accident and emergency department management of deliberate self-poisoning. *Br J Psychiatry* 1988; **152:** 830-3.

12 O'Dwyer FG, D'Alton A, Pearce JB. Adolescent self-harm patients: audit of assessment in an accident and emergency department. *BMJ* 1991; **303:** 629-30.

13 Royal College of Psychiatrists. *The General Hospital Management of Adult Self-Harm. A Consensus Statement on Standards for Service Provision.* London: Royal College of Psychiatrists, 1994.

14 Platt S, Hawton K, Kreitman N, Fagg J, Foster J. Recent clinical and epidemiological trends in parasuicide in Edinburgh and Oxford: a tale of two cities. *Psychol Med* 1988; **18:** 405-18.

Variations in clinical experience of pre-registration house officers: the effect of London

Thomas Dent*, MRCP, Senior Registrar in Public Health Medicine, Cambridge and Huntingdon Health Commission, Fulbourn Hospital, Cambridge CB1 5EF, **Jonathan Gillard**, MB, Clinical and Research Fellow, Division of Neuroradiology and Department of Neurology, The Johns Hopkins Hospital and University School of Medicine, Baltimore, Md 21287, USA, **Emma Aarons**, MRCP, Registrar in Infectious Diseases, Regional Infectious Diseases Unit, North Manchester General Hospital, Manchester M8 6RB, and **Penelope Smyth-Pigott**, Assistant Federation Secretary, British Postgraduate Medical Federation, 33 Millman Street, London WC1N 3EJ.

Keywords: Pre-registration house officers; education; clinical experience; London; Thames regions.

Health Trends 1995; **27**: 22-6

Summary

A postal questionnaire was used to examine possible differences in clinical experience of pre-registration house officers (PHROs) in eight former English regions, and, within the Thames regions, between teaching hospitals, and non-teaching hospitals in Inner London, Outer London and outside London.

The main measurements were the numbers of patients clerked in an average week as emergency, routine or day admissions or as outpatients; the number of patients under the respondents' care at time of reply; the experience of specific clinical conditions gained; the overall adequacy of clinical experience; and the suitability of posts for preparing respondents to work as casualty officers, senior house officers, or general practitioners.

The results indicate that less clinical experience was aquired by PRHOs training in the Thames regions. They had fewer admissions per week, fewer patients, and exposure to fewer surgical conditions. Within the Thames regions, there was a gradient of improving educational quality (in all areas of this study) from the teaching hospitals, through the non-teaching hospitals in inner and in outer London, and then to the hospitals outside London. No differences were found between Thames region posts outside London and non-Thames regions.

Introduction

British medical graduates undergo a year's training in pre-registration house officer (PRHO) posts approved for this purpose by their university, before full registration with the General Medical Council (GMC) allows them to take up posts providing more specialised training. The quality of their training depends in part on the clinical experience their posts provide. McManus et al showed that the experience gained by clinical students trained in London was less than those trained elsewhere in Britain[1], and house officers at London teaching hospitals see fewer patients, perform more inappropriate tasks, and are less

*Correspondent: Dr T Dent

satisfied with their clinical training than those elsewhere[2]. We analysed data from the second British Postgraduate Medical Federation House Officer Survey, to examine training provided at hospitals in different parts of England, and we examined differences within the Thames regions.

Methods

A postal questionnaire was sent to PRHOs in the former Thames regions (London and the surrounding counties), and four other geographically and demographically representative former regions (East Anglia, Mersey, Northern and Wessex). We wrote to all house officers in the first seven regions, and to a randomly selected sample of 95 of the 175 house officers in the former Wessex region, a total sample size of 1,670; Wessex was sampled because several recent questionnaires on other topics had already been undertaken - and we chose not to burden them further.

The survey took place in December 1992 and January 1993 (detailed elsewhere)[3]. The questionnaire requested information about the respondents' medical school; the number of patients under their care; the number clerked in an average week as emergency, routine or day admissions, or as outpatients; the frequency of patients with various clinical conditions; and the suitability of the clinical experience provided. Respondents were also asked the numbers of patients clerked in quiet and busy weeks - these results are not given here, but the question may have reduced any exaggerations for an average week. Copies of the questionnaire are available from the authors. Data analysis was by Students t-test, analysis of variance, Pearson's χ^2-test, the Mann-Whitney U-test and the Kruskal-Wallis H-test. The significance of p-values was adjusted for multiple tests using a Bonferroni-corrected nominal p-value of 0.00179.

Results

We received 1,146 returned questionnaires, a response rate of 69%. Regional response rates lay between 68% and 73%, apart from Mersey (53%) and Wessex (80%). Not all respondents answered every question.

Comparison between regions

The numbers of patients clerked weekly are shown in Table 1. The differences between regions for emergency, day and total

Table 1: *Numbers of patients clerked weekly by house officers and under house officers' care in eight regions*

Region	Median (inter-quartile range) of weekly admissions					Median (inter-quartile range) of patients under house officers' care	Number of respondents
	Emergency	Routine	Day	Outpatient	Total		
East Anglia	12 (10-20)	6 (2-12)	2 (0-5)	0 (0-0)	23 (19-31)	22 (16-28)	84
Mersey	10 (6-14)	6 (2-12)	5 (0-9)	0 (0-1)	22 (14-32)	22 (16-28)	98
Northern	10 (8-15)	6.5 (2-15)	4 (0-8)	0 (0-0)	25 (17-34)	20 (15-29)	160
Wessex	12 (9-15)	6 (3-10)	2 (0-4)	2 (0-5)	22 (17-28)	20 (15-28)	76
North-East Thames	8 (5-10)	5 (3-10)	1 (0-4)	0 (0-2)	15 (11-23)	15 (11-23)	216
North-West Thames	10 (5-12)	5 (2-10)	0 (0-5)	0 (0-1)	18 (12-24)	17 (12-24)	175
South-East Thames	10 (7-14)	6 (2-10)	1 (0-5)	0 (0-0)	19 (13-26)	17 (12-24)	190
South-West Thames	10 (6 -12)	5 (2-11)	3 (0-6)	0 (0-1)	20 (14-30)	20 (15-25)	144

Significant a posteriori comparisons using Mann-Whitney U-test (adjusted p < 0.05):

Number of admissions:
Emergency: East Anglia with Mersey and all Thames regions; Wessex with North-East and North-West Thames; Northern with North-East and North-West Thames; South-West Thames with North-East Thames; South-East Thames with North-East Thames.

Routine: nil.

Day: North-West Thames with Mersey, Northern and South-West Thames; North-East Thames with Mersey, Northern and South-West Thames; South-East Thames with Mersey and Northern.

Outpatient: nil.

Total: North-East Thames with all regions except North-West and South-East Thames; North-West Thames with all non-Thames regions; South-East Thames with Northern and East Anglia.

Numbers of patients under house officers' care in eight regions:
All Thames regions except South-West Thames with East Anglia, Mersey and Northern; Wessex with North-East Thames; South-West Thames with North-East Thames.

Table 2: *House officers' clinical experience scores and reported acquisition of clinical experience in eight regions*

Region	Clinical experience scores		Acquisition of clinical experience					
	Median (inter-quartile range) House physicians	House surgeons	Gaining about the right amount of clinical experience No.	%	Seeing too few patients to gain sufficient clinical experience No.	%	Seeing so many patients that there is no time to learn No.	%
East Anglia	49 (45-53)	37 (33-40)	55	67	4	5	22	27
Mersey	43 (36-50)	35 (32-39)	40	42	6	6	45	47
Northern	46 (42-51)	35 (32-37)	100	64	11	7	42	27
Wessex	51 (46-54)	34 (31-36)	53	72	1	1	19	26
North-East Thames	45 (39-51)	34 (29-37)	139	64	41	19	29	13
North-WestThames	45 (41-49)	34 (29-37)	82	47	48	28	40	23
South-East Thames	47 (42 -51)	32 (30-35)	112	61	24	13	45	24
South-WestThames	48 (45-53)	34 (30-37)	96	68	10	7	35	25

The clinical experience score was derived from the list of clinical conditions (see appendix) by assigning one point to "never", two to "once" and so on, and then summating.

Significant a posteriori comparisons using Mann-Whitney U-test (adjusted p < 0.05):

House physicians: Wessex, East Anglia and South-West Thames with Mersey, North-West Thames and North-East Thames.

House surgeons: East Anglia with North-East, North-West and South-East Thames.

Table 3: *Suitability of post for training in eight regions*

Region	Casualty officer			General practitioner			Senior house officer in specialty		
	Mean	SD[1]	No.	Mean	SD[1]	No.	Mean	SD[1]	No.
East Anglia	2.82	0.96	83	2.77	1.09	82	2.36	1.03	80
Mersey	3.19	1.09	97	3.00	1.04	95	2.92	1.16	97
Northern	3.30	1.06	153	2.73	1.04	151	2.64	1.07	152
Wessex	2.92	0.87	75	2.51	0.86	74	2.30	0.90	74
North-East Thames	2.81	1.05	209	2.89	1.07	211	2.61	1.16	208
North-West Thames	2.93	1.04	174	2.90	1.02	173	2.83	1.02	172
South-East Thames	2.99	1.03	184	2.89	1.09	187	2.67	1.05	185
South-West Thames	2.84	1.08	142	2.73	1.08	142	2.57	1.09	142

[1] Standard deviation

Scores on a scale from 1 [very suitable] to 5 [very unsuitable].

Significant a posteriori comparisons using Scheffé's test (p < 0.05):

Casualty officer: Northern with North-East Thames and South-West Thames.

clerkings are significant (Kruskal-Wallis H: χ^2 = 80.6, p < 0.0001; χ^2 = 42.1, p < 0.0001; χ^2 = 72.3, p < 0.0001 respectively). House officers in the Thames regions have significantly fewer admissions in all categories (Mann-Whitney U: emergency p < 0.0001, routine p = 0.0077, day p = 0.0001, outpatient p = 0.016, total p < 0.0001).

The numbers of patients under house officers' care also vary significantly between regions (Kruskal-Wallis H: χ^2 = 67.0, p < 0.0001) (Table 1). House officers in the Thames regions have significantly fewer patients (medians 17 versus 20, Mann-Whitney U: p < 0.0001).

House officers were asked how often they had seen various common medical and surgical conditions (see appendix) - never, once, two to four times or more than four times. A score was derived by assigning one point to "never", two to "once", and so on (Table 2). The variation between regions is significant (Kruskal-Wallis H: medicine χ^2 = 46.4, p < 0.0001, surgery χ^2 = 22.0, p = 0.0026), although only for surgery is there a significant difference between Thames and non-Thames regions (Mann-Whitney U: p = 0.0004). The clinical experience score proved relatively insensitive, as most PRHOs had seen most of the listed conditions more than four times.

Table 2 shows house officers' subjective views of the clinical experience - there are significant differences between regions (χ^2 = 105, p < 0.0001).

House officers were asked to assess the suitability of their post for preparing them to work as a casualty officer, a general practitioner (GP) and a senior house officer (SHO) in the appropriate specialty (Table 3). Mean scores differed between regions for training as a casualty officer and an SHO (one-way ANOVA: p = 0.0002; p = 0.0007 respectively) but not as a GP (p = 0.051). Thames house officers were less likely to view their posts as suitable for training casualty officers (t-test: p = 0.001).

Comparisons within the Thames regions
Hospitals in the Thames regions were classified as teaching (Charing Cross, Guy's, King's, Middlesex, Royal Free, Royal London, St Bartholomew's, St George's, St Mary's, St Thomas', University College and Westminster) and non-teaching. Non-teaching hospitals were divided into inner London (within the North/South Circular Road), outer London and non-London.

The numbers of emergency patients, day patients and the total number of patients varied significantly between teaching and non-teaching hospital (Kruskal-Wallis H: p < 0.0001, p = 0.0002, p < 0.0001 respectively), with a trend for fewer patients being

Table 4: *Numbers of patients clerked weekly by house officers and under house officers' care in the Thames regions*

Type of hospital	Median (inter-quartile range) of weekly admissions					Median (inter-quartile range) of patients under house officers' care	Number of respondents
	Emergency	Routine	Day	Outpatient	Total		
Teaching	7 (4-10)	6 (3-10)	0.5 (0-4)	0 (0-1)	14 (11-20)	15 (10-20)	186
Inner London	8 (5-12)	5 (2-8)	0.5 (0-4)	0 (0-2)	15 (11-22)	16 (12-20)	108
Outer London	9 (6-13)	5 (2-8)	2 (0-6)	0 (0-1)	19 (13-28)	18 (13-25)	136
Non-London	10 (8-15)	5.5 (2-10)	0 (0-6)	0 (0-0)	21 (15-30)	20 (15-25)	261

Significant a posteriori comparisons using Mann-Whitney U-test (adjusted p < 0.05):

Emergency: Teaching with Outer and Non-London; Inner London with Non-London.

Routine: Nil.

Day: Teaching with Outer and Non-London.

Outpatient: Nil.

Patients under house officers' care: Teaching with Outer and Non-London; Inner London with Non-London.

Table 5: *House officers' clinical experience scores and reported acquisition of clinical experience in the Thames regions*

Type of hospital	Clinical experience scores		Acquisition of clinical experience					
	Median (inter-quartile range)		Gaining about the right amount of clinical experience		Seeing too few patients to gain sufficient clinical experience		Seeing so many patients that there is no time to learn	
	House physicians	House surgeons	No.	%	No.	%	No.	%
Teaching	42 (38-48)	30 (25-34)	78	44	66	37	32	18
Inner London	45 (42-49)	33 (30-36)	74	70	14	13	17	16
Outer London	47 (44-52)	35 (31-38)	80	60	18	13	35	26
Non-London	48 (42-51)	35 (32-37)	175	68	22	9	57	22

The clinical experience score was derived from the list of clinical conditions (see appendix) by assigning one point to "never", two to "once" and so on, and then summating.

Significant a posteriori comparisons using Mann-Whitney U-test (adjusted $p < 0.05$):

House physicians: Teaching with Outer and Non-London.

House surgeons: Teaching with all others.

seen at teaching hospitals, and inner London hospitals (Table 4). House officers tend also to have fewer patients under their care at these hospitals (Table 4, Kruskal-Wallis H: $p < 0.0001$), which is corroborated by differences in the amount of clinical experience reported by house officers at different types of hospital (Table 5) (Kruskal-Wallis H: house physicians $p < 0.0001$, house surgeons $p < 0.0001$). Respondents also differ in the proportions believing they have too few patients, enough patients or too many patients (Table 5) ($\chi^2 = 68.4$, $p < 0.0001$). There is a trend, from non-London hospitals to teaching hospitals, for an increasing proportion of house officers to report too few patients (χ^2 for trend = 49.1, $p < 0.0001$). House officers' views on the suitability of their posts for training also show differences between types of hospital (Table 6) (one-way ANOVA: $p < 0.0001$ for all three training objectives).

Discussion

House officers' training in the eight former English regions appears to vary substantially, with marked differences between Thames and non-Thames regions. Those training in the Thames regions acquire less clinical experience than those training elsewhere. Their posts provide fewer admissions per week, fewer inpatients, and exposure to a smaller number of surgical conditions. Thames house officers are more likely to say that they are seeing too few patients to gain adequate clinical experience, and less likely to say that they are seeing too many to learn properly. Some of our questions sought subjective responses, but the similar pattern seen in those, and questions with objective answers, suggests that some inferences can be drawn.

Most problems occur in London; Thames house officers outside London gave responses similar to those from non-Thames regions. Within the Thames regions a similar pattern is seen, with more clinical experience available away from teaching hospitals and inner London. More than one-third of house officers in teaching hospitals think that they are seeing too few patients - in particular they perceive their posts as offering poor training, contrary to the perceived value of a teaching hospital post.

Optimum clinical experience for house officers has not been defined, and it could be argued that those in the Thames regions are receiving a satisfactory amount. The GMC has previously set 30 as a maximum number of inpatients[4]: 7% of Thames house officers exceeded this, compared with 12% of non-Thames house officers. The 1992 guidance does not set a maximum number of inpatients[5], but the Committee of Postgraduate Deans[6] endorsed the original GMC recommendation that the number of inpatients should be between 10 and 30. Some 83% of the workload of Thames and non-Thames house officers lay within these limits; 9% of Thames respondents had less than 10 patients compared with 5% of non-Thames respondents. The Thames house officers' replies show that they themselves believed their jobs were too quiet. After five months of work, 4.2% of teaching hospital house physicians had not seen a patient with myocardial infarction, compared with 1.5% of those in the Thames regions outside London; 10% of house surgeons at teaching hospitals had not seen a patient with appendicitis, compared with 2.5% in the Thames regions outside London.

Table 6: *Suitability of post for training in Thames regions*

Type of hospital	Casualty officer			General practitioner			Senior house officer in specialty		
	Mean	SD[1]	No.	Mean	SD[1]	No.	Mean	SD[1]	No.
Teaching	3.28	1.00	181	3.36	1.01	185	3.11	1.00	182
Inner London	2.89	1.07	103	2.65	1.00	108	2.50	1.15	103
Outer London	2.81	1.07	134	2.86	0.96	135	2.65	1.04	133
Non-London	2.71	1.04	257	2.65	0.91	253	2.45	1.05	255

[1] Standard deviation

Scores on a scale from 1 [very suitable] to 5 [very unsuitable].

Significant a posteriori comparisons using Scheffé's test ($p < 0.05$):

Casualty officer, general practitioner and senior house officer in specialty: Teaching with all others.

Appendix: *List of clinical conditions in survey questionnaire*

Medicine
Myocardial infarction
Cerebrovascular accident
Drug overdose
Pulmonary oedema
Lobar pneumonia
Gastro-intestinal haemorrhage
Meningitis
Pneumothorax
Exacerbation of chronic obstructive airways disease
Diabetic keto-acidosis
Hypoglycaemia
Severe asthma
Renal failure
Liver failure
Subarachnoid haemorrhage
Status epilepticus

Surgery
Appendicitis
Pancreatitis
Gallstone disease
Bowel obstruction
Colorectal carcinoma
Breast carcinoma
Head injury severe enough to warrant admission
Multiple injuries
Ruptured aortic aneurysm
Ischaemic leg
Gastro-intestinal haemorrhage

These differences compound those reported by McManus *et al*[1]. They found that London-trained medical students accumulated less clinical experience than those who trained elsewhere. Many London students undertake training as house officers in London, and therefore may have less experience by the end of the pre-registration year.

Conclusion

Pre-registration house officers should consider the educational opportunities that different hospitals offer.

Acknowledgements

We are grateful to the house officers who completed our questionnaire, to the clinical tutors and their staff who distributed it; to Prof John Anderson and Prof Peter Flute and Dr Trevor Bailey, Dr John Biggs, Dr Michael Nicholls, Dr Hugh Platt, Dr Elizabeth Shore and Dr Jack Tinker who gave us permission to survey in their Regions; to Julie DeSimon who co-ordinated the fieldwork, to Professor Chris McManus for advice and to Dr R C King who inspired these projects. We are also grateful to Mr Julian Lipscombe for data entry.

This project was funded by the South-East Thames Dean of Postgraduate Medicine.

References

[1] McManus IC, Richards P, Winder BC, Sproston KA, Vincent CA. The changing clinical experience of British medical students. *Lancet* 1993; **341:** 941-4.

[2] Dent THS, Gillard JH, Aarons EJ, Crimlisk HL, Smyth-Pigott PJ. Pre-registration house officers in the four Thames regions: II. comparison of education and workload in teaching and non-teaching hospitals. *BMJ* 1990; **300:** 716-8.

[3] Gillard JH, Dent THS, Aarons EJ, Smyth-Pigott PJ, Nicholls MWN. Pre-registration house officers in eight English regions: a survey of quality of training. *BMJ* 1993; **307:** 1180-4.

[4] General Medical Council. *Recommendations on general clinical training.* London: GMC, 1987.

[5] General Medical Council. *Recommendations on general clinical training.* London: GMC, 1992.

[6] Committee of Postgraduate Deans. *The pre-registration experience: implementing change.* London: COPMED, 1994.

Job satisfaction and health of house officers in the West Midlands

Caron Grainger*, MFPHM, Senior Registrar in Public Health Medicine, **Eleanor Harries**, PhD, Research Fellow, **John Temple**, FRCS, Postgraduate Dean, and **Rod Griffiths**, FFPHM, Professor of Public Health Institute of Public and Environmental Health, The University of Birmingham, Birmingham B15 2TJ.

Keywords: Pre-registration house officers; Occupational Stress Indicator; job satisfaction; stress; mental and physical ill-health.

Health Trends 1995; **27**: 27-30

Summary

A postal questionnaire survey was conducted in 1993 to determine the job satisfaction and current state of health of British-trained pre-registration house officers (PRHOs) working in the West Midlands Regional Health Authority. The questionnaire included parts of the Occupational Stress Indicator looking at job satisfaction, and mental and physical ill-health (as manifestations of stress). Out of 234 eligible PRHOs 182 (78%) returned questionnaires: female PRHOs had significantly higher scores for physical and mental ill-health than male PRHOs; 14.2% of PRHOs had scores for mental ill-health, and 17.6% scores for physical ill-health that were higher than the average reported for patients with psycho-neurotic disorders. The PRHOs had significantly lower scores for all individual aspects of job satisfaction and total job satisfaction, and significantly higher scores for mental and physical ill-health than a comparative group of junior hospital doctors (all grades), and a large group of non-health-care white-collar workers. These results indicate that there is a need to raise awareness of stress and stress-related problems faced by junior doctors, and to provide adequate support.

Introduction

Much has been written about the causes and effects of stress in a medical career[1,2,3], but little is known about these factors in the first year of professional life, nor the possible after-effects in future years[3]. Nonetheless, there is now considerable evidence to suggest that doctors, and junior doctors in particular, are stressed. Measurements for stress such as alcohol abuse/dependency[4,5], and suicide[6] are higher for doctors than the general population - examples of this are a 72% greater risk of suicide and a 77% higher risk of dying from cirrhosis of the liver among doctors compared with the general population[4].

Job satisfaction and levels of mental and physical ill-health are related to stress[7], and research shows a relation between mental and physical health and job satisfaction and sickness absence[8,9]. The consequences of these relationships may include low morale and motivation, poor communication, faulty decision-making, and poor relationships with colleagues and with patients - all might affect patient care. Stress is costly for the employer, and stress-related illnesses may be responsible for more absenteeism from work than any other cause[9]; the annual costs to British

*Correspondent: Dr C Grainger

industry of absenteeism through anxiety and depression have been estimated to be £5.3 billion (1991 costs)[10].

Besides concerns about the state of morale and the effects of stress upon doctors, it is reported that between 18 and 25% of doctors leave the main public sector within 5 years of graduation[11]. This includes doctors who are taking time out for domestic reasons, practising medicine abroad, or outside of the NHS (eg armed forces). It is estimated that a small proportion of doctors cease practising medicine all together[12,13] - doctors are an expensive resource, and their loss is financially wasteful; it has been estimated that the cost of training each new doctor is around £158,500 (£188,000 including an intercalated degree) (*BMA News Review*, October 1993). As a result of reports such as these, the West Midlands Regional Board of Postgraduate Medical and Dental Education agreed to fund a study looking into the morale of pre-registration house officers (PRHOs) across the West Midlands Region.

Method

All 294 PRHOs working within the West Midlands Regional Health Authority were surveyed. The postal survey questionnaire comprised two parts - one looked at biographical data, issues related to medical training, and coping behaviour/lifestyles such as smoking, drinking and exercise; subjects were asked to quantify their average alcohol and tobacco consumption, and their amount of exercise. The second part was taken from the Occupational Stress Indicator (OSI)[14], and dealt with job satisfaction and well-being.

The questionnaire was piloted on three separate occasions, on 75 PRHOs, at the Queen Elizabeth Medical Centre in Birmingham, and at the Queen's Medical Centre in Nottingham. The pilot studies revealed that most questionnaires were never received by their intended recipient (usually lost in the doctors' mess/internal mail), and so the distribution process was changed to distribution by clinical tutors. Questionnaires were distributed to all PRHOs employed within the West Midlands in March 1993 (one month after the start of the PRHOs' second house job), and returned direct to one of the authors (EH) by freepost. Three recalls were undertaken: by clinical tutors to all PRHOs, and by two further telephone recalls to non-responders only. Questionnaires were coded for the second and third recall, and were therefore not anonymous - but the codes were only known to one of the authors (EH) who was not in a position to influence the careers of the responders. Confidentiality of individual data was assured in the questionnaire itself, the covering letter, and during telephone recalls.

Fourteen people from the sample population were involved with the pilot testing of the questionnaire, and were excluded from further analysis. In addition, one of the PRHOs issued with a questionnaire was in fact a SHO, and one PRHO never took up post - these were also excluded, along with 44 PRHOs who were trained outside the UK (excluded because foreign doctors may have additional stress factors which might bias the results). The survey population therefore consisted of 234 people.

Measures - the Occupational Stress Indicator (OSI)
Data were collected from each respondent on their health (mental and physical ill-health, as manifestations of stress) and job satisfaction. These were calculated from the OSI scales[14], a reliable and validated instrument[15] which has been used successfully in the health care setting[8,9,16,18].

The health scale comprised two sub-scales measuring mental and physical ill-health, by use of six-point Likert-type scales of symptom frequency. The mental ill-health scale took account of a range of cognitive aspects of strain, whilst the physical ill-health scale looked at somatic symptoms of anxiety and depression (eg sleep and appetite disturbances). The physical health scale measures somatic manifestations of mental ill-health.

The overall job satisfaction score was produced from five sub-scale scores (the absolute range values in brackets):

Achievement value and growth looks at perceived opportunities for advancement, how valued they feel, and whether their job is rewarding (6-36)

Job itself measures satisfaction with the type of work (4-24)
Organisational design and structure looks at how well the organisation functions (5-30)

Organisational processes looks at perceptions of whether the organisation facilitates or hinders getting things done (4-24)

Personal relationships examines views about the quality of personal relationships at work (3-18)

Normative data for the OSI used for comparison included a group of junior doctors of all grades[8] (n=40) (PRHO to senior registrar); and a large group of non-health-care blue and white collar workers (n=6326)[16]. Data on hospital consultants and GPs was available, but not considered appropriate for comparison.

Results
One hundred and ninety six doctors (83.3%) responded to the survey, of which 182 (78%) have been used for this analysis - the remaining 14 questionnaires were answered selectively, and were excluded. This response was comparable with other studies of junior doctors[2].

The respondents had a mean age of 24.5 years (SD 1.73); 85 (47%) were men and 96 (52.7%) were women (one respondent did not answer the question); 144, (79.1%) were caucasians, the remainder being Indian (18, 9.9%), Pakistani (4, 2.2%), Chinese (6, 3.3%) or another race (7, 3.6%).

Table 1: *Job satisfaction and health scores for West Midlands PRHOs*

	Males (n=85)	Females (n=96)
Achievement value and growth (range 6-36)	19.35 (4.33)	19.33 (94.19)
Job itself (range 4-24)	14.05 (2.87)	13.84 (2.77)
Organisational structure and design (range 5-30)	14.57 (3.53)	15.07 (2.97)
Organisational processes (range 4-24)	12.89 (3.56)	12.95 (3.44)
Personal relationships (range 3-18)	10.67 (2.17)	10.99 (2.43)
Total job satisfaction (range 22-132)	71.55 (13.45)	72.06 (12.73)
Mental ill-health (range 18-108)	57.73 (14.57)	65.19 (13.17)[1]
Number of cases	9	16
Physical ill-health (range 12-72)	31.19 (10.60)	36.28 (10.74)[1]
Number of cases	11	20

[1] p<0.001 (t test)

Job satisfaction and health
There were no significant differences between the scores for job satisfaction for men and women PRHOs, however, women had significantly higher scores for mental and physical ill-health, as manifestations of stress, shown in Table 1. Rees and Cooper[9] also found women to have significantly higher scores for stress-related physical ill-health, and Jick and Mitz[17] reported women to show significantly higher psychological stress symptoms than men.

People with clinically significant mental health problems can be identified by comparing their scores with those of patients with psycho-neurotic disorders. The critical scores for mental ill-health are 76.97 or above, and for physical ill-health are 45.39 or above[18]. Against this criteria, 26 PRHOs exceeded the mental ill-health scores, and 32 exceeded the physical ill-health scores. 15 people exceeded both scores (6 men and 8 women, one unknown).

These results agree with other studies reporting higher levels of stress and depression in women doctors compared to men doctors[1,2,19], and could be attributed to the increased pressures (stressors) which they encounter, for example, lack of women role models; prejudice from patients, and conflict between work and personal roles[20].

Job satisfaction was associated negatively with mental ill-health (r = -0.3859 p<0.001) and physical ill-health (r = -0.4062 p<0.001) - also found by Rees and Cooper[9].

Ethnicity
For the purposes of comparison, respondents were classified as caucasian or non-caucasian, and there were no significant differences in any aspect of job satisfaction, total job satisfaction, or mental and physical ill-health.

Lifestyle behaviour
There was no correlation between those drinking in excess of the recommended amounts of alcohol (14 units per week for women, 21 units per week for men), smoking, or taking less than one hour of exercise per week and those who exceeded the ill-health scores, for either physical or mental ill-health.

Discussion
West Midlands PRHOs had significantly lower scores for all aspects of job satisfaction, and significantly higher scores for mental and physical ill-health when compared with a small sample of junior doctors nationally, (n=40; Table 2). This difference may be due to the differences in seniority and age between the two groups because the junior doctors group does not consist solely of PRHOs. A positive relation has been reported between age and job satisfaction in physicians[21]. Reuben[22] observed a fall in prevalence of depressive symptoms in house officers with successive years of training, and suggested several possible explanations for this: occupational and personal changes; a decrease in the number of hours worked; a decrease in the least satisfying aspects of patient care (eg. clerking work); and an increase in skills and confidence. Hsu and Marshall reported similar observations[19].

Table 2: *Comparison of mean scores for West Midlands PRHOs with those of junior hospital doctors in Manchester Health Authority, and Occupational Stress Indicator (OSI) normative data on non-health care workers*

	Survey (n=182)	Junior doctors (n=40)	OSI normative data (n=6326)
Achievement value and growth (range 6-36)	19.32 (4.24)	22.78 (4.44)[1]	21.66 (5.74)[1]
Job itself (range 4-24)	13.92 (2.81)	15.84 (2.39)[1]	16.34 (3.25)[1]
Organisational structure and design (range 5-30)	14.82 (3.24)	17.27 (3.02)[1]	16.73 (4.17)[1]
Organisational processes (range 4-24)	12.91 (3.48)	15.49 (2.87)[1]	15.54 (3.78)[1]
Personal relationships (range 3-18)	10.81 (2.32)	11.84 (1.98)[1]	11.78 (2.51)[1]
Total job satisfaction (range 22-132)	71.74 (13.05)	83.22 (11.22)[1]	81.76 (16.64)[1]
Mental ill-health (range 18-108)	61.78 (14.32)	55.30 (12.25)[1]	56.54 (12.25)[1]
Physical ill-health (range 12-72)	34.03 (11.08)	28.35 (8.29)[1]	29.69 (9.79)[1]

[1] p<0.001 (t test)

Our results for job satisfaction appear to accord with the general feelings PRHOs are reported to hold about their work. Dowling and Barrett [3] reported that a large part of the house officers' work is seen as the 'dogsbody role', where they carry out repetitive clerical and administrative tasks, and act as continuity people who fill gaps in hospital services, and ensure that the pace of admissions is maintained.

Table 3: *Current initiatives in the West Midlands*

1 A counselling and stress management service, open to all hospital doctors and dentists in training

2 The introduction of a 'Stress Survival Guide', a short booklet describing the symptoms of stress and some techniques for managing it. A section of the guide gives specific details of sources of help.

3 A 'How to be an effective house officer' course, open to all final year medical students, will begin in May 1995. This runs over two days, and looks at the practicalities of entering employment e.g. time management, finances, self care etc. rather than the management of clinical situations.

The survey population also had significantly lower scores for all aspects of job satisfaction, and significantly higher scores for mental and physical ill-health when compared with the normative occupational stress indicator data (Table 2). People working in health care settings experience higher levels of occupational stress, and as a consequence perhaps have lower levels of job satisfaction and higher levels of mental and physical ill-health. Rees and Cooper[8] also reported that their group of health care workers reported higher levels of mental and physical ill-health, and lower levels of job satisfaction compared with a population of non-health workers.

We, like others[23,24], believe that the prevention of stress-related disorders requires intervention at both organisational and individual level. Examples of current initiatives to raise awareness of stress and stress related problems, and to provide support to doctors within the West Midlands are shown in Table 3. Additionally, there appears to be a need to make additional support available to female PRHOs, for example by providing information about part-time training and advising on careers in which family life can be sensibly combined. As the 'New Deal' is implemented for junior doctors and hours of work are reduced[25], the effect of the changes upon the welfare of doctors will need to be investigated. If reducing hours of work leads to higher pressures during duty hours, stress levels may not be reduced.

Conclusion
The results of this study indicate that PRHOs in the West Midlands are in need of support in order to improve job satisfaction and to reduce the physical and mental ill-health manifestations of stress.

Further details of the work, including copies of the questionnaire can be obtained from the authors.

Acknowledgements
We thank NFER-Nelson for their permission to reproduce sub-scales taken from the Occupational Stress Indicator, and the clinical tutors across the West Midlands for their help in distributing the questionnaires, and the Regional Board of Postgraduate Medical and Dental Education for funding the work.

References
1 British Medical Association. *Stress in the medical profession.* London: BMA, 1992

2 Firth-Cozens J. Stress in medical undergraduates and house officers. *Br J Hosp Med* 1989; **41**: 161-4.

3 Dowling S, Barrett S. *Doctors in the making - the experience of the pre-registration year*. Bristol: University of Bristol School for Advanced Urban Studies,1991.

4 Office of Population Censuses and Surveys. *Occupational mortality 1979-80, 1982-3*. London: HMSO, 1986.

5 Balarajan R. Inequalities in health within the health sector. *BMJ* 1989; **299:** 822-5.

6 Richings JC, Khara GS, McDowell M. Suicide in young doctors. *Br J Psychiatr* 1986; 1**49:** 475-8.

7 Cooper CL, Sloan SJ, Williams S. *Occupational Stress Indicator Management Guide*. Windsor: NFER-Nelson,1988.

8 Rees DW, Cooper CL. Occupational stress in health service employees. *Health Serv Man Res* 1990; **3:** 163-72.

9 Rees D, Cooper CL. Occupational stress in health service workers in the UK. *Stress Medicine* 1992; **8:** 79-90.

10 Confederation of British Industry/Department of Health. *Promoting mental health at work*. London: Department of Health, 1991.

11 Medical Manpower Standing Advisory Committee. *First Report. Planning the medical workforce*. London: Department of Health, 1992.

12 Parkhouse J. *Doctors careers. Aims and experiences of medical graduates*. London: Routledge, 1991

13 Nicholl JP. *A profile of doctors who recently deregistered. Final report to the Department of Health*. Medical Care Research Unit, University of Sheffield 1990

14 Cooper CL, Sloan SJ, Williams S. *Occupational Stress Indicator 1988*. Windsor: NFER-Nelson, 1988.

15 Robertson IR, Cooper CL. The validity of the Occupational Stress Indicator. *Work and Stress* 1990: **4:** 29-39.

16 Cooper C, Sloan SJ, Williams S. *Occupational Stress Indicator Data Supplement*. Windsor: NFER-Nelson, 1989

17 Jick TD, Mitz LF. Sex differences in work stress. *Academy of Management Review* 1985; **10(3):** 408-20.

18 Cooper CL, Sloan SJ, Williams S. *Occupational Stress Indicator Data Supplement*. Windsor: NFER-Nelson, 1993

19 Hsu K, Marshall V. Prevelence of depression and distress in a large sample of Canadian Residents, Interns and Fellows. *Am J Psych* 1987; **144(12):** 1561-6.

20 Firth-Cozens J. Sources of stress in women junior house officers. *BMJ* 1990; **301:** 89-91.

21 Linn LS, Yager J, Cope D, Leake B. Health status, job satisfaction, job stress and life satisfaction among academic and clinical faculty. *JAMA* 1985; **254:** 2775-82.

22 Reuben DB. Depressive symptoms in medical house officers - effects of training and work rotation. *Arch Intern Med* 1985; **145:** 286-8.

23 Johnson WDL. Predisposition to emotional distress and psychiatric illness amongst doctors: the role of unconscious and experiential factors. *Br J Med Psychiatr* 1991; **64:** 317-29.

24 Thapar A. Psychiatric disorder in the medical profession. *Br J Hosp Med* 1989; **42:** 480-3.

25 Department of Health. *Hours of work of doctors in Training: the new deal*. London: Department of Health, 1991. (Executive Letter: EL(91)82).

A note from the Editor

Readers should note the comments of the Chairman of the Editorial Board on Page 3 of this issue. Over 90% of papers submitted for consideration for publication are rejected. A recurring problem is that many of the papers we receive are not in the required format - mostly papers not following the research style of **Summary**, **Introduction**, **Method**, **Results**, **Discussion** and **Conclusion**. At present, unsolicited reviews or editorials are published by exception. Authors are also reminded that studies involving patients or their records require Local Research Ethics Committee (LREC) approval, or some formal proof that LREC approval was not required - self-declaration by the author(s) is in general not sufficient. With these particular points in mind, potential authors are reminded to take note of the Guidelines for Authors which are set out below.

Guidelines for authors

Submission of papers:

Topics for inclusion in *Health Trends* should, in general, be related to medical aspects of National Health Service practice, management, planning, implementation, and evaluation. Original contributions from a variety of disciplines are welcome and must be submitted exclusively to *Health Trends*. The readership is general and international; authors should therefore avoid 'jargon' terms or concepts used by a particular specialty or country. Papers are accepted for publication on their scientific originality and general interest and on the understanding that they will be subjected to editorial revision. Papers and accompanying material will not be returned to authors unless specifically requested.

All papers accompanied by a covering letter containing the signature of all co-authors, should be submitted to the Editor at the address shown on the inside front cover of the Journal. The original paper and four copies are required to facilitate the editing and review process, and, where appropriate, the research questionnaire should accompany the paper. All papers will be acknowledged, and authors will be notified of a paper's accceptance or rejection once the review process is complete. A reference number will be given for enquiries and *must* be quoted in any communications with the Medical Editorial Unit. *Papers based on research involving patients/clients including their records should indicate in the text that the research had the prior approval of the appropriate ethics committee.*

Referees:

Papers accepted for consideration will be reviewed independently by a panel of referees to include referees from: the Editorial Board; expert referees; a statistician from the Department of Health (DH) and/or the Office of Population Censuses and Surveys; the relevant DH Policy Division; and the Editors. The referees are asked their opinion on the originality, scientific reliability (with emphasis on methodology), clinical importance (where relevant) and overall suitability for publication. The Editor retains ulimate responsiblity.

Presentation of Papers:

Authors are strongly advised to examine a copy of *Health Trends* for examples of Journal style, expression and lay-out. Information must be presented succinctly without being telegraphic. Normally, papers should not exceed 2,000 words, or contain more than six tables. The paper should be typed in double spacing, on one side only of A4 paper, with a margin of at least three centimetres all round using standard typewriter typeface of Courier 10 pitch. The first page of the paper must contain the full title of not more than eight words, a list of keywords that clearly describe the sbject matter of the article, and the author'(s) name(s) with one forename for each author Each author should indicate his/her professional discipline, current appointment and one degree or qualificaiton. Each page should be numbered consecutively. Quotation marks in the text must be single, except where a statement is a direct quotation, when double marks should be used. Authors should keep at least one copy of their paper for reference. The paper should indicate the person to whom proofs and enquiries are to be sent, their full address (including postal code), a telephone and FAX number, and the name of a co-author (if applicable) who can provide information to the Editorial Unit when the correspondent is unavailable.

Summary:

A summary of not more than 200 words should follow the title page and must contain information on the problem, subjects, methods, findings and conclusions. This paragraph should précis the major points in such a way that it can be read independently. No references should appear in the summary.

Headings:

Papers should follow the usual convention, ie title page; keywords and sumary; introduction; method; results; discussion; conclusion; acknowledgements; references; tables and figures. Major headings should be in **bold** (dark type, lower case lettering (initial capitals only) starting at the left-hand margin. Minor headings (sub) should be typed in the same way and underlined. Headings should not be numbered.

Data and terminology:

All quantitative measurements should be in terms of the International System of Units (SI), but blood pressure should continue to be expressed in mm Hg. All drugs and other compounds should be referred to by their accepted generic names, and not by their proprietary names, unless it is essential for clarification purposes. Statistical methods should be defined, and any not in common use should be described in detail or supported by references. Where percentages are given within the text and tables, the actual number of patients/clients on which these are based should also be provided.

Abbreviations:

When first used in the text, a term which the author wishes to abbreviate must be spelt out in full, with its abbreviation in brackets. Thereafter, the abbreviation alone should be used. Abbreviations should be in capitals and unpunctuated, eg Health Education Authority (HEA).

Tables:

Tables accompanying papers should be identified by Arabic numerals, typed in double spacing on separate sheets of paper (ie not incorporated within written text), and contain only horizontal lines. Authors should indicate an appropriate position within the text for tables and/or figures. The title of the table should be brief, but the contents should contain a clear and complete explanation of what the data represent (the kind of objects enumerated and how they have been categorised in the tables; the geographical and time coverage; and units of measurement; and the source(s) of the data). Footnotes should be used sparingly, but included where necessary, to clarify the data and to give a fuller descripton of compact headings. Data contained in the tables should be simple and supplement, not duplicate, information in the written text. Wherever possible, all figures used in tables, containing data or derived statistics should be rounded to the nearest whole number. Columns and rows should be arranged in some natural order of size.

Figures:

Figures should leave the reader in no doubt about the kind of objects, events, people or measurements represented; the units used; the geographical coverage; the time period covered; the scale of measurements; the source(s) of the data; and how to interpret the chart. This information should appear around the edge of the chart, in the heading, in a label on the axis, or, if necessary, in a clear key. Figures should be completely lettered, the size of the lettering being appropriate to that of the drawing. Headings should be typed using double spacing. Any material previously published, or unpublished, should be accompanied by the wrtten consent of the copyright holder; full acknowledgement and references must be given.

Graphs:

Graphs should be presented as clear line drawings on white paper or graph paper. Data used to determine value 'points' indicated must accompany all graphs.

References:

The accuracy and completeness of references are of the utmost importance, and are the authors' responsibility. A maximum of 10 key references per paper should be numbered consecutively in the order in which they appear in the text. At the end of the paper, a full list of references, presented in Vancouver style, should give the names and initials of all the authors (unless there are more than six, when only the first three should be given followed by *et al*). Authors' attention is drawn to the further reading section of these Guidelines which provides full guidance.

Acknowledgements:

Only those who have made substantial contribution to the study and/or preparation of the paper should be acknowledged. The sources of grants, equipment and drugs should be included. Authors should obtain permission from people acknowledged by them, as readers may infer their endorsement of the data and conclusion published.

Resubmission of papers:

When papers are returned to authors with referees' comments for revision, the revised paper should be submitted with an accompanying letter describing the action taken concerning each point made by the referees. If any change suggested is not thought appropriate, the reason should be clearly explained. Floppy disks preferably in Wordperfect 5.1 should be enclosed where available.

Correspondence:

Letters must relate directly to recently published articles, and must be limited to a maximum of 450 words. Letters will also be submitted for reviewers' comments. The Editor reserves the right to edit all correspondence, and to decide if, and when, correspondence should be published. Letters must be signed by all the authors.

Publication process:

An edited version of the paper will be sent to authors for their comments/approval prior to publication. The page-proofs will then be sent by FAX (or post) to the corresponding author who is responsible for checking the type-setting accuracy *thoroughly* and giving written consent for publication. Alterations to the text are strongly discouraged at this stage, and in general only essential updating amendments will be accepted.

Offprints

Twenty offprints can be supplied to the corresponding author, providing the request is made to the Editorial Unit before the paper is submitted for printing. However, authors should note that HMSO charge for this facility.

The Editor and Unit staff welcome written or telephone contact with authors who have any queries or suggestions.

References

[1] Department of Health. *Local Research Ethics Committees*. Heywood (Lancashire): Department of Health, 1991. (Health Service Guidelines: HSG(91)5).

Further reading

[1] International Committee of Medical Journal Editors. Uniform requirements for manuscripts submitted to biomedical journals. *BMJ* [Clin Res] 1988; **296**: 401-5.

[2] International Committee of Medical Journal Editors. Uniform requirments for manuscripts submitted to biomedical journals. *BMJ* [Clin Res] 1982; **284**: 1766-70.

[3] Guidelines for writing papers. *BMJ* [Clin Res] 1989; **298**: 40-42.

[4] Chapman M, Mahon B. *Plain figures*. London: HMSO, 1986.